Healthy Ageing and Longevity

Volume 1

Series editor

Suresh I.S. Rattan, Aarhus, Denmark

More information about this series at http://www.springer.com/series/13277

Katarina Friberg Felsted · Scott D. Wright

Toward Post Ageing

Technology in an Ageing Society

Springer

Katarina Friberg Felsted
Scott D. Wright
Gerontology Interdisciplinary Program
College of Nursing
University of Utah
Salt Lake City, UT
USA

ISBN 978-3-319-09050-4 ISBN 978-3-319-09051-1 (eBook)
DOI 10.1007/978-3-319-09051-1

Library of Congress Control Number: 2014944545

Springer Cham Heidelberg New York Dordrecht London

Printed on acid-free paper

Springer is part of Springer Science+Business Media (www.springer.com)

Foreword

It is possible to make two predictions about the United States, indeed, all advanced industrialized countries, between now and, say, the year 2035. First, the pace of technological change will continue, as manifested in telecommunications, medical science, military technique, and so on; second, populations will grow older: that is, median age will rise as the number of older adults increases and the number of children declines. The first of these trends will come about because of investments in research and development already in place. The second will come about because those over age 65 have already been born and fertility rates have been falling worldwide. Note that prediction of a rapidly "ageing society" does not depend on further gains in life expectancy or medical miracles. It simply reflects the growing proportion of elders compared to other age groups. In sum, we can discern many elements of "the shape of things to come" already: namely, an ageing society influenced by rapid changes in technology. It is because of this forecast that Felsted and Wright's book has such enormous importance.

We need make no judgment about whether society will be better or worse off because of anticipated changes in demography and technology. On the one side, there are those who fear for the future of an older society on a global basis. Consider the title of Ted Fishman's book *Shock of Grey: The Ageing of the World's Population*: "How it Pits Young Against Old, Child Against Parent, Worker Against Boss, Company Against Rival, and Nation Against Nation." On the other side, there are voices of optimism about population ageing, though less prominent than the pessimists. For example, Laura Carstensen, *A Long Bright Future*, with its full title: "Happiness, Health and Financial Security in an Age of Increased Longevity."

Similarly, we are familiar with optimistic pictures based on technology, whether in computers and telecommunications or advances in the biology of ageing. On this last point, we may cite Aubrey de Grey, editor of the journal *Rejuvenation*, who believes we could be on the threshold of dramatic changes in maximum human lifespan. He joined Ray Kurzweil, who predicts a "singularity" of man-machine interaction akin to science fiction. There are also those who look at the same trends, but forecast a gloomy shape of things to come: for example, Bill

Joy's much discussed article "Why The Future Doesn't Need Us." In short, with technology, as with demography, there have always been utopian and dystopian visions of the shape of things to come.

In truth, we are in no position now to make specific forecasts about breakthroughs in science and technology that could alter the shape of the human lifespan itself: e.g., de Grey's notion that humans could live to be 500 or 1,000 years old. This kind of "inflection point" (in the phrase used in this book) is conceivable, but we have no way of estimating its probability. Even if we avoid speculating about de Grey's scenario, we can conduct a thought experiment and imagine, say, the discovery of an "Alzheimer's vaccine," which would end that burden in later life. Similarly, we could imagine breakthroughs in regenerative medicine to allow more people to live up to the empirical maximum lifespan (120 years). Successfully these domains are conceivable, though I offer no predictions about probability in either case. But we can imagine near-term scenarios that deserve consideration.

I put forward two contrasting scenarios for an ageing society in 2067 in my article on "Reflecting on the 21st Century." I offered two different pictures of the next half-century, one very optimistic, and one very pessimistic. What is needed today is a sustained examination of the interaction between technology and demography, not to make predictions, but to better understand what is already happening. Let me offer a few examples. Smart phone technology, along with email, has already altered the delivery of home health care. Most would regard that as a good thing: e.g., homebound elders on Skype with their grandchildren. But expanded access to telecommunications could accelerate financial elder abuse as older people with more assets become victims through computer technology. Consider another example. Success in life-preserving medical technology could enable more people to survive life-threatening conditions. But life-preserving technology can also enable those with advanced dementia or other debilitating conditions to survive beyond the time they would wish to live.

Thus, technology typically turns out to be a two-edged sword: i.e., unanticipated problems along with hoped-for benefits. The real point of these examples of telecommunications and biomedical technology is that we do not need to wait for a distant future to see mixed results. We already live in a world of rampant financial elder abuse, mediated by telephones and email, and we already live in a world where we speak about a "right to die" to defeat the ever-encroaching force of medical technology in maintaining biological life. Thus, it is critical for us to examine this intersect of technology and philosophy.

The authors of this book urge us, properly I think, to reflect on the possibility of "transcending ageing," of living in a "post-ageing" world. But something of this sort has already been happening. When we hear slogans like "Sixty is the New Forty," what we are reminded of is that the experience of old age—say, of people 65 years of age and older—is already very different than what it was until recently, and so we find ourselves in an inflection point. In the first place, there are more elders, not primarily because of advances in medical technology, but because of public health measures, falling fertility rates, and an ageing Baby Boom. The real income of elders is higher than in the past, and their options and choices are different. Let me cite two modest examples from the 40 years I have been in gerontology. Forty years ago, mandatory retirement was not illegal. Forty years ago, there was no such thing as Elderhostel (now Road Scholar) or other opportunities for lifelong learning. Forty years ago, elders had substantial rates of poverty, rates which have now dropped to the point approximating other adult age groups. "Old age" today looks very different than it did when I (now 69) entered the field of ageing. We may not have entirely created a "post-ageing" world but we have already begun to see elements of that world, which is precisely why the issues discussed in this book are so important.

Those who look at technology tend to invoke images of hope or fear, and those who look at ageing, individual or societal, have their own hopes and fears. There is a modest academic literature about the future of population ageing but serious assessment of technology and the future of ageing remains to be done. Pessimists have captured public attention, perhaps in part because of widespread ageism criticized by geriatricians like Robert Butler and John Rowe. It is exactly on this point that the study of technology and ageing can make a contribution: not by predicting a specific path (e.g., an Alzheimer's vaccine) that may or may not ever happen. Instead, reflection on technology and ageing, as we see in this volume, can help us recover a more vigorous "sense of the possible," or to use the terms of Castoriadis, a "social imaginary" so critically needed to counter the pessimism and ageism that still remain widespread. This vigorous sense of the possible does not require us to become utopian cheerleaders for technology as the solution to all problems of ageing. Nor does it permit us to surrender to the pessimism too often heard from cultural critics. Rather it requires us to have a sense of an open future, a future not entirely predictable or foreshortened. And, most importantly, it offers us the possibility of realistic hope, needed today more than ever.

Harry R. Moody
Santa Barbara

Acknowledgments

To my parents, Birgitta and Stig, beacons of older adult generativity, who never for a moment made me think I was anything but capable. To my sister, Anna-Karin, who is more precious than an eye.

To my interdisciplinary academic colleagues, both local and national, for their emulable examples. To my mentors, Dr. Caserta and Dr. Wright, for their sustained illumination.

To my children, Logan, Christian, and Bennett, who tolerated this book as if it were a new sibling, and generously made consequential adjustments and allowances. And to my husband, Pat—for his unfailing encouragement and full support.

Katarina Friberg Felsted

After 30 years of academic service in the field of gerontology, I would like to acknowledge the deep legacy through their publications and writings of these scholars: Glen Elder, Bernice Neugarten, Urie Bronfenbrenner, Robert Kastenbaum, Andrew Achenbaum, Harry R. Moody, and Thomas R. Cole—who offered profound inspiration and motivation in my academic training to think, discover, and most importantly to philosophically question the received view of the ageing experience and to reflect on the ageing experience in creative ways. I would like to especially highlight the role of Thomas R. Cole and his scholarship on the history of ageing and humanistic gerontology as transformational in my perspectives of the ageing experience as placed in the context of time and cultural milieu.

I also would like to thank Dr. Dale Lund for his supportive mentorship and establishing an academic environment at the University of Utah for bold ideas and allowing gerontology to be truly interdisciplinary. I want to thank my colleague Katarina Friberg Felsted for her professional focus and determination in leading the way in the publication of this work and for being an integral part of the scholarship from the beginning with a symposium at the Gerontological Society of America on philosophical issues of technology and ageing.

I dedicate this book to my two sons—Logan and Ian Wright. The emergence and impact of technology will be fully realized in their life course and ageing experience—and for the many generations to follow.

Scott D. Wright

Contents

Part II Toward Post Ageing: A Critical Examination and Provisional Typology for Understanding the Varied Roles of Technology in an Ageing Society

Abstract

In this work, the authors present a provocative interdisciplinary meta-analysis (contrasting "paradigms" with "inflection points") to describe and understand the emergent and expanding role of technologies that hold both promise and possible peril for transforming the ageing process in this century. This book is directed to professionals who wish to review the continuum of varied constructs and intersects of technologies ranging from those purporting to enhance the "activities of daily living" in older adults, to those that would enable the older worker to stay "competitive" in the labor market, to those who propose to extend longevity, making senescence negligible, ultimately claiming to transcend "ageing" itself—moving toward a transhumanistic domain. There is a discussion of the points and counterpoints of technological advances that would influence a reconstruction of what it means to "age" when embedded in a post-human vision for a post-biological future. While these advancements and intersects represent indicators of "optimal ageing" they may in fact represent the desire and resultant actions that would transcend 'ageing' altogether. It is proposed that society has reached critical mass in both literature and technological outcomes, and therefore, we can begin to address the actual, putative, and speculative impacts and influences on the ageing experience. Based on this proposition, it is further claimed that advances in technology would affect epistemological and ethical issues and alter the expectations and educational practices for the ageing experience in our lifetime.

Part I
Transcending Disciplinary and Paradigmatic Tensions in Gerontology

Chapter 1
The Use of Inflection Points

Abstract In brief, inflection point [1.0]—representing the *Philosophy of Ageing* as a technique for coping with the shortness of life, or the finiteness of time—has been superseded by several new inflection points, with [5.0]—representing *Post Ageing,* or ageing as an *artifact,* with an array of bio-technological advancements and interventions in the ageing process as our current temporal setting. Between these two diametrical poles, one quite philosophical and one quite technological, there have been three other *inflection points* ([2.0], [3.0], and [4.0]). Each *inflection point* represents a change in direction in the flow of purpose and praxis for what constitutes a dominant theme in conducting inquiry relating to ageing. Many readers will find the heuristic of *inflection points* to be closely related to other terms that have been used in the history and philosophy of science, such as *paradigms, conjectures, exemplars, disciplinary matrix*, and the *cognitive apparatus* of a given scientific community (Conant and Haugeland 2000; Kuhn 1970, 1977; Popper 1963; Suppe 1977). Similarly related has been the use of terms like *research programme, research tradition, representational spaces, critical transitions* and *threshold of epistemologization* (Agamben 2009; Hung 2001; Lakatos 1970; Laudan 1984; Scheffer 2009).

Keywords Life expectancy · Ageing experience · Ageing process · Ageing research · Gerontology · Social gerontology · Gerontological theory · Paradigm · Heuristic · Inflection points · Conceptual framework · Philosophy · Demographics · Optimal ageing · Post ageing · Theoretical model · Technologies

1.1 The Use of *Inflection Points* in the Explanation and Understanding of Scholarship for the Ageing Experience

> We are in the midst of two striking trends: widespread population ageing and rapid diffusion of technology. Both phenomena are very new in human history (Charness 2004) (p. xxv).

K.F. Felsted and S.D. Wright, *Toward Post Ageing*,
Healthy Ageing and Longevity 1, DOI 10.1007/978-3-319-09051-1_1

The assumed trajectory of the journey of life has changed dramatically in terms of both life *expectancy* and life *outlook* over the centuries. Sophocles captured the "fundamental impermanence of the natural and constructed world" via the play Oedipus at Colonus. Here is Oedipus talking to Theseus in what is arguably his greatest speech (Sophocles 2005, translation by Costa),

> Dearest son of Aegeus, none but the gods
> Escape old age and death; all else
> Time in its relentless flood sweeps away.
> The strength of earth and body fades… (p. 14).

The great flux of life as precursor to one's mortality was also the purview of the Roman Stoics. Both Marcus Aurelius and Seneca offered their philosophical perspectives on the seemingly brief span of time that was life. Their viewpoint was that life only appeared to be short as humans were apt to take for granted the time that was given. Here, Seneca's thoughts *On the Shortness of Life* (translation by Costa 2005),

> Life is long enough and a sufficiently generous amount has been given to us for the highest achievements it if were all well invested. But when it is wasted in heedless luxury and spent on no good activity, we are forced at last by death's final constraint to realize that it has passed away before we knew it was passing. So it is: we are not given a short life but we make it short, and we are not ill-supplied but wasteful of it. (pp. 1–2)

And Marcus Aurelius (translation by Gill 2013), the philosopher-king, from his work *Meditations*,

> Altogether the interval is small between birth and death; and consider how much trouble, and in company with sort of people and in what feeble body this interval is laboriously passed. Do not then consider life is a thing of any value. For look to the immensity of time behind thee, and to the time which is before thee, another boundless space. In this infinity then what is the difference between him who lives three days and him who lives three generations? (p. 268)

Marcus Aurelius emphasized the quality of life over the quantity of life as he persuasively indicated that having a longer period of time to be alive would not necessarily make for a better life. But that was then, and this is now.

Obviously much has changed in our current understanding of the human condition and the ageing experience since Seneca's time and the Roman world. In hindsight, an observer can posit that we have experienced significant transitional phases in our understanding of the journey of life. These epochal transitions have critical implications for the study of the ageing process. One of the primary goals of this book is to create a new conceptual approach to the macro-level phases of scholarship for the study of ageing. But before we elaborate on that proposed heuristic, let us examine some traditional understandings of transitional developments in the comprehension of the human condition.

One example of such a transitional design would be the supposed perennial division found between the humanities (*Geisteswissenschaften*) and the natural sciences (*Naturwissenschaften*) which has produced two modes of knowing: *Verstehen* (understanding) and *Erklären* (explanation) (Rickman 2004; Schmidt 2006).

This differentiation is related to the perspectives of Snow (1964) and his influential, albeit controversial, publication addressing the breakdown of communication between the "two cultures" of modern society, science and the humanities. Since Snow's publication there have been attempts to integrate the two domains (Brockman 1995; Wilson 1998) or at least better articulate why there are differences between them (Gay 2010). Some see the division as counterproductive and many have argued persuasively for the humanities to appreciate more contributions from the natural sciences, particularly research on human cognition, creating an integrated approach to culture and the human condition (Kagan 2009; Lehrer 2009; Slingerland 2008). Another example is the perennial debate and discussions of consciousness that surround the seeming incommensurability with human subjective experiences and an objective world and the resulting monist (idealism vs. materialism) and dualist theories (i.e., Cartesian dualism) (Blackmore 2004; Ramachandran 2004). Another example of such transitions is the distinction of and emphasis on *vita contemplativa* in contrast to *vita activa* (following Arendt 2013). The transition from *vita contemplativa* to *vita activa* also heralded the emergence of the modern scientific enterprise, which (*contra* Arendt) would now be considered the world-immanent epistemological measure of knowledge and understanding (Brient 2001). It appears that the enterprise of *science* is how we primarily focus our theories and methods on the ageing experience as well.

The historical development of gerontology as a discipline, as interdisciplinary, a taxonomy, an approach, a lexicon, and as a profession has a checkered and dendritic course of progression, and many have attempted to profile the major events and prevailing streams of philosophy and thought along the way (Achenbaum 1995, 2009; Bass and Ferraro 2000; Cole 1992; Hendricks and Achenbaum 1999; Katz 1996). Although many gerontologists would concede that the "scientific management of ageing" (Cole 1992) is the prevailing paradigm in which most of the research and policy in ageing is derived, there are also several who would contest this hegemony and would seek equitable awareness to perspectives that lie outside the foundational scientific enterprise, such as in the humanities and in critical gerontology (Cole et al. 2010; Biggs et al. 2003; Bengtson et al. 2009). Here is Katz (1996) arguing for the "undisciplining" of gerontology because of the rich sociocultural dimensions of the ageing experience,

> Ageing and old age are intrinsic to every form of knowledge and cultural practice: spiritual, ritual, mythical, symbolic, artistic, metaphorical, and architectural. They are the central organizing resources for a multitude of social structures from nomadic pastoralism to complex kinship systems to state like bureaucracies. Indeed, ageing and old age have been so diversely and richly understood that no single knowledge of them is universal. Nor should it be. The meanings of ageing and old age are scattered, plural, contradictory, and enigmatic. They are confirmation that the mysteries of age have furnished the human imagination with limitless opportunities to express itself. Age, is everywhere, but the world's cultures have taught us that age has no fixed locus. (p. 1)

As Bengtson et al. (2005) have indicated in their concise chapter, "Are theories of ageing necessary?", published in Johnson's *The Cambridge Handbook of Age and Ageing,* the perspectives from constructivist and critical orientations offer an alternative to the precepts of science (or more specifically—positivism). While, for the most part, the business of gerontology is in the scientific business, Bengtson et al. (2005) lament the lack of theory driven research and practice in gerontology (see also Alley et al. 2010; Powell 2009),

> The field of gerontology has accumulated vast amounts of data over the past decades, creating a goldmine of potential theoretical knowledge. Yet explicit theory development has lagged—prompting some to observe that gerontology remains data-rich and theory poor (Bengtson et al. 2005, p. 4; see also Bengtson and Schaie 1999).

Bengtson et al. (2005) acknowledge the role of critical theory and social construction perspectives but nevertheless acknowledge that "science remains the reigning paradigm" (p. 17), and then go further by specifically stating that the "biomedicalization of ageing remains a guiding research paradigm" (p. 6). This assessment also appears to be a reactionary stance by several others (primarily within the sub-domain of the social sciences) who either fear the dominion of the biomedical sciences or the slippery slope of scientism and/or reductionism (Bengtson et al. 1999; Biggs et al. 2003; Katz 2003). Ferraro (2000) has gone on record as an editor of the *Journal of Gerontology: Social Sciences* hoping to make gerontology more inclusive, yet also stating that because "health issues are inextricably related to the ageing process...gerontology flirts with being medicalized" (p. S3).

The debate and dialogue continues in multiple dimensions and directions in terms of gerontological theory, methodology, and practice (Alkema and Alley 2006; Alley et al. 2010; Bass and Ferraro 2000; Bengtson et al. 2009; Ferraro 2006; Haber 2009; O'Donohue 1992). Some see the potential for a "unified theory" (the holy grail) and an "integrative model" within social gerontology (Bass 2006, 2009), while others ponder if the "age-specific" status of gerontology is in post-mortem when placed in the context of "life course" conceptual models (Settersten 2006). There are also the on-going academic and paradigmatic tensions between life course sociology and life span psychology (Baltes and Nesselroade 1984) that bring to bear different levels of foci and analyses (micro vs. macro) of the human condition and ageing experience. Recent attempts have been made to find where the different pathways may complement one another by "extending the interrogation" and establishing common ground in a potential integrated paradigm or the proposal of a new paradigm altogether (Dannefer and Daub 2009; Diewald and Mayer 2009; Settersten 2009). While it appears that there is much to be worked out in this regard, we did find Settersten's (2009) comments about how the behavioral and social sciences need to engage more directly and extensively with the biological and medical sciences to be highly relevant to the goal of this book. We completely agree with Settersten's call for a deeper integration of the human sciences with those of the natural sciences in investigating the vagaries of human development. As you will soon discover, we are proposing that the domain of digital technologies and bio-technologies will also become a major cross-cutting influence in the explanation and understanding of the ageing experience (Critser 2010; Cutler 2005, 2006; Read et al. 2008). But we noted some troubling statements by Settersten regarding "reductionistic tendencies" in such domains as genomics and neurosciences. Settersten's (2009) concerns seem to raise the specter of fear that conducting science at the molecular level would somehow leave out the human spirit and that only molar level analyses could capture the essential nuances of the "ageing experience."

This categorization and distinction setting appears to be rebuilding a wall between *Geisteswissenschaften* and *Naturwissenschaften* or between *Verstehen* and *Erklären* when it comes investigating to the ageing experience. In other words, raising the flag of "reductionism" for relatively new foci of analyses (i.e., genomics and neurosciences) appears to resurrect the "two cultures" when approaching the ageing experience. This unfortunate stance would mean that the potential for interdisciplinary theory-building (Bass 2009; Bengtson et al. 2009) and vertical integration through many levels of inquiry could stall because of the belief that "meaning" or "making connections" for the ageing experience is the domain of *only* the behavioral and social sciences. In other words, "extending the interrogation" would only be allowed to go so far—perhaps between sociology and psychology—but deeper vertical connections with the biomedical sciences or biotechnological aspects would not be worthy of further pursuit for fear of creating an academic slippery slope toward *consilience* (Wilson 1998), or a level of reductionism that would exclude the study of what makes us "human." Biggs et al. (2003) have claimed that exchanges with humanities and social sciences "have been met with indifference" by the biomedical sciences (Biggs et al. 2003, p. 5) and Katz (2003) believes that "critical gerontology" has been marginalized due to "the predominance of biomedically-driven funding policies" (p. 26). This kind of bickering and academic tension is understood when defending the academic territories and safe-guarding the heterogeneity of perspectives for the ageing experience (Bass 2009) but it may also reinforce the parceling out of the study of ageing to a predetermined set of specialties deemed to be appropriately only understood or researched at one level, be it cognitive or biological or psychological. In other words, we end right back where we started with disciplinary territories (or home departments) that are marked by rigid silos of specialists talking to one another in their appointed domains of either macro- or mid-range or micro-level theories and methods. The study of ageing is then left to "specialists" who defend their hallowed space either out of academic loyalty or career construction (Bass 2009; Hendricks and Achenbaum 1999).This kind of strategic enterprise cannot be good for the investigation of and about the full spectrum of the ageing condition.

Fortunately, the second edition of the *Handbook of Theories of Ageing* (Bengtson et al. 2009) has made great strides to be more inclusive and integrative with a substantive awareness of the dividends of interdisciplinary theory building and research (Bass 2009). Nevertheless, the desire to identify an embryonic paradigm is bound to be problematic within a realm that either claims to be interdisciplinary or is the subject of many separate disciplines claiming their own paradigmatic identities.

While we could debate the nuances of life-span psychology and life course sociology as to the best approach to ageing phenomena, and we could discuss intricacies of whether gerontology is really a full-fledged discipline, multidisciplinary, or interdisciplinary, and whether gerontology is best served by fully developing theories or by primarily focusing on application, practice, or policy (Bengtson et al. 2005), we think it is best to proceed by examining the progress of the "gerontological imagination" (Bass and Ferraro 2000; Wilmoth and Ferraro 2007) *not* as a paradigm per se but through an alternative conceptual model. Using a pre-theoretical structure helps us see what the inclusive activities in our scientific enterprise, ideology, and practice are being *driven by* and *leading towards* in the domain of ageing. The usage, definition, and application of the word "paradigm" in gerontology/ageing have been highly challenging. It is questionable whether or not there is "one" paradigm that actually exists in gerontology:

> Gerontology has dramatically increased its intellectual capital; however, one limitation of its propitious growth is the perceived absence of a paradigm: the fundamental image that a discipline has of its subject matter…Especially in scientific fields, a paradigm establishes a general set of organizing principles that provides coherence or maps the field. A paradigm also defines what should be studies. (Bass and Ferraro 2000, p. 99)

Although we agree with the basic assumptions of how a paradigm generally operates according to Bass and Ferraro (2000), we also believe, in contrast, that any meta-theoretical shifting with the "gerontological imagination" (Bass and Ferraro, 2000) should to stay clear of the epistemological baggage that is carried along with the discourse on Kuhnian (that is, Thomas Kuhn) based paradigms. The notion of a monolithic, eminent paradigm does not seem applicable to gerontology if we assume it to be multi or interdisciplinary; however, Bass and Ferraro (2000) have indicated that gerontology may be best understood as "a multiple-paradigm science" (p. 99), or perhaps there may be a paradigm (i.e., "gerontological imagination") but in a "latent or embryonic form" (p. 100). We submit that this only complicates matters, especially when placed in context with the Kuhnian conceptualization of a paradigm as it relates to the philosophy and history of science.

Thus, following in the tradition of Cole (1992) and others (e.g., Achenbaum 1995; Bass and Ferraro 2000; Hendricks and Achenbaum 1999; Katz 1996), we are taking the "long view" in proposing an overarching interpretation—*a heuristic* (Gigerenzer 2008; Wimsatt 2007)—of the primarily 20th century developments in the scientific enterprise associated with the field of ageing that led to the establishment of an *Weltanschauung* in the field of ageing. The use of heuristic methods has a rich history (Groner et al. 1983) and continues to have modern applications (Wimsatt 2007). The basis of using a heuristic approach ("inflection point" vs. "paradigm") in this manuscript is proposed to be an effective, satisfactory, and "fast and frugal" strategy for creating a deductive pedagogical platform by which we can address a vast inventory of published work in the domain of the study of ageing. The heuristic is deliberately used to indicate an incomplete and unconfirmed system, yet, it is still a deductive approach to the selected nodes and exemplars ("fast and frugal") that represent the inflection points, nevertheless, the end result—the outcome—of five proposed inflection points is offered as an acceptable, satisfactory and reasonable discovery for understanding the history and development of major trends in gerontology over the course of several decades. Our use of inflection points and the corresponding exemplars is grounded in the notion of "bounded rationality," and more specifically, the approach of *satisficing* (Gigerenzer et al. 2002). Our goal was to balance quality and quantity in terms of the analysis and synthesis of relevant nodes of literature and thus when embedded within an "ecological rationality" (Gigerenzer 2008), we are careful to note that our proposal of inflection points is not based in any Bayesian decision-making design, or algorithm or multiple linear regression model with all possible parameters measured and quantified. Yet, we assert that a careful examination of the literature can lead to a robust interpretation of major trends and patterns in gerontology and that the use of inflection points is more satisfying and reasonable than the use of paradigms in our field.

But we also propose that the existing world view will soon be supplanted by another emergent world-view or conceptual framework in the 21st century. It is proposed that this new world view will have the capacity to transform the epistemology of gerontology and ontological concerns for ageing individuals for decades to come. We further claim that this superseding shift represents what we call (and heuristically use to examine such meta-theoretical transitions)—an *inflection point.*

1.2 The Use of Inflection Points Versus Paradigms in Gerontology

We propose that there have been several key *inflection points* in understanding our modern journey of life as ageing individuals. We use the term "inflection point" as the preferred label—and as a heuristic strategy—to understand and organize the sequential but inter-related epistemological and ontological shifts that are associated with the study of the ageing process. By "inflection points," we are referring to the mathematical concept that signifies a point on a curve at which the sign of the curvature for a function changes direction (Weisstein 2009; see Fig. 1.1).

Points of inflection, derivatives, second derivatives (i.e., derivative of the derivative), and *curvature* are terms used in the modeling of dynamical systems to describe and measure rates of change (i.e., derivative) for biological phenomena (Adler 2012; see also Scheffer 2009), but are used here deliberatively as a heuristic (Marsh et al. 2004; Roberts 2004; Wimsatt 2007) and a hermeneutic (Schmidt 2006) in the investigation of scholarship in the field of ageing. When used specifically in the domain of modeling life dynamics, a function with a positive derivative is one that is *increasing* and one with a negative derivative is one that is

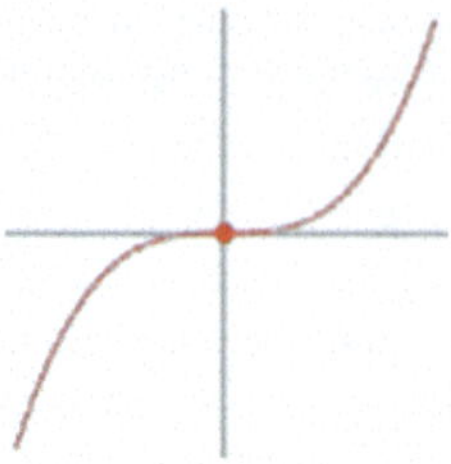

Fig. 1.1 Inflection Point Heuristic (Also inspired by http://en.wikipedia.org/wiki/Inflection_point)

decreasing. Furthermore, the second derivative tells whether the graphical interpretation of the function curves upward or downward (Adler 2012).

This is used to assess the rate of growth (and interest) in the scholarship on ageing as either *increasing* or *decreasing* (as a function of point in time) depending on the prevailing stream of thought in the majority of research, teaching, and practice in the field of ageing within a designated point in time. One major caveat for the use of this device is that there is *no* actual mathematical algorithm used to determine or create an actual graphical outcome for the analysis of determining inflection points; rather, the graphical image serves to create the heuristic (see Marsh et al. 2004) by which we might understand the transitions in both focus and primary activities associated with research and application in the field of ageing. We are careful here to avoid the cavalier poaching of scientific terms from other disciplines (especially from mathematics), especially given the critiques of Sokal and Bricmont (1998) who have found many abuses of science in the "postmodern context" where there is haphazard and promiscuous use of extrapolation of ideas from the natural to the social sciences. But just as Dawkins (2009) used the same strategy in his book, *The Greatest Show on Earth*, by taking the liberty of borrowing a concept (i.e., "theorem"—although Dawkins did change it slightly to "theorum") from mathematics to create his heuristic of a *scientific theorum* in explaining the role of evolutionary theory in the context of scientific facts, we will take the liberty of borrowing *one term* that has relative cross-disciplinary relevance. We propose that the use of this terminology can help to advance a new viewpoint and perspective to understand the change, growth and transitions of gerontological scholarship without the necessity of falling back to the notion of the Kuhnian paradigm and the attendant assumptions of that historical framework for interpreting scientific activity in our field. Thus, one major point of departure (interpreted as necessary) when using this heuristic rather than the traditional term of "paradigm" (via Kuhn) is to understand and appreciate the interconnections among various inflection points over time that are *not* necessarily diminished or dropped even after a new inflection point has emerged.

In fact, each proposed inflection point is intimately tied to and connected to the previous one. Within gerontology, we do not find an existing era of "normal science" to be in essence incommensurable and mutually exclusive to the following one after a significant revolution has occurred. In addition, in contrast to the supposed Copernican-like "revolutions" and subsequent puzzle-solving of normal science of Kuhnian paradigms, we propose that there are subtle incremental shifts, and although shifts do occur and new directions are forged, they are not like the decisive breaks that Kuhn envisions—as though the research traditions in gerontology have behaved like the shockwaves of plate tectonic movements. In other words, we would propose that there is *not* the sense of a "scientific revolution" within the field of gerontological scholarship as Kuhn rendered it with a sense of a "clean break" from previous operating paradigms,

> … discoveries that cannot be accommodated within the concepts in use before they were made. In order to make or to assimilate such a discovery one must alter the way one thinks about and describes some range of natural phenomena. (Kuhn 2000, p. 14–15)

Rather it is proposed here that to better understand the changes in the prevailing stream of thought and purpose we name them *inflection points*, indicating a shift in direction for the major themes in scholarship over a designated period of time. Inflection points do have some similarities with what Sherraden et al. (2001) refer to as "pretheoretical tensions" in the field of gerontology (especially as it relates to "productive ageing"), but inflection points carry a longer and deeper historical perspective for our field both in retrospect and prospectively.

To place this in perspective, we propose that there have been five major inflection points in the extant history of gerontological scholarship and practice (see Table 1.1).

In brief, inflection point [1.0]—representing the *Philosophy of Ageing* as a technique for coping with the shortness of life, or the finiteness of time—has been superseded by several new inflection points, with [5.0]—representing *Post Ageing,* or ageing as an *artifact*, with an array of bio-technological advancements and interventions in the ageing process as our current temporal setting. Between these two diametrical poles, one quite philosophical and one quite technological, there have been three other *inflection points* ([2.0], [3.0], and [4.0]).

Each *inflection point* represents a change in direction in the flow of purpose and praxis for what constitutes a dominant theme in conducting inquiry relating to ageing. Many readers will find the heuristic of *inflection points* to be closely related to other terms that have been used in the history and philosophy of science, such as *paradigms, conjectures, exemplars, disciplinary matrix*, and the *cognitive apparatus* of a given scientific community (Conant and Haugeland 2000; Kuhn 1970, 1977; Popper 1963; Suppe 1977). Similarly related has been the use of terms like *research programme, research tradition, representational spaces, critical transitions* and *threshold of epistemologization* (Agamben 2009; Hung 2001; Lakatos 1970; Laudan 1984; Scheffer 2009). But our preference for using *inflection points* within gerontological scholarship is based on four substantive motivations:

(1) There are inherent complications that have followed the Kuhnian historiography of science and its attendant terminology of *paradigms, normal science, crisis, gestalt switches, conversion experiences, revolutions,* and the highly

Table 1.1 Inflection points: directional shifts in prevailing theme in gerontology/ageing

[1.0]: Philosophy of ageing (Ageing as a *reflection*)
[2.0]: Bio-medical diseases of ageing (Ageing as a *problem*)
[3.0]: Demographics of ageing (Ageing as a *challenge*)
[4.0]: Optimal ageing (Ageing as a *reward*)
[5.0]: Post ageing (Ageing as an *artifact*)

debatable and contentious notion of *incommensurability between paradigms* (Agamben 2009; Boghossian 2006; Caneva 2000; Mayo 1996; O'Donohue 1993; Radder 1997; Shapin 2010; Sokal and Bricmont 1998; Tauber 2009; Von Dietze 2001).

(2) The use of paradigm to describe scientific advancements via normal and revolutionary science may not be applicable to *all areas* of study in science (Carvalho 2006; Mayr 1994).

(3) The concept of paradigm and its operational definitions varies across disciplines even when paying homage to its Kuhnian origination. For example, O'Donohue (1993) challenged the use of Kuhnian paradigms for the field of psychology, and Bhopal (1999) argued for a pro-active use of the Kuhnian notion of paradigm to advance common themes in textbooks in the field of epidemiology and public health; Weaver and Olson (2006) discussed four different "paradigms" for use in nursing research; and Weaver and Olson (Ferrario et al. (2008) see "successful ageing" as a requisite paradigm in changing nursing students' attitudes about ageing (see also Dillaway and Byrnes 2009). Kaye et al. (2003) suggested an alternative frame of reference, "toward a productive ageing paradigm" for geriatric practice, while Weaver (1999) envisions gerontology education as a "new paradigm for the 21st century", offsetting ageism and building intergenerational unity by focusing on successful/productive ageing as opposed to geriatric health and social problems. Chapin and Cox (2001) argue for a more "strengths-based and empowerment-oriented paradigm" of practice in social work, which sounds very much like Haber's call (2009) to add an "empowerment paradigm" to the field of gerontology because of the changing ageing demographics associated with baby-boomers. Carpi et al. (2008) use the term *paradigm* to carve out a new domain of "post-reproductive genetics" in relation to human longevity evolutionary biology due to the "peculiar" findings in this specialty. It is obvious from these few examples that the Kuhnian concept of paradigm has been used to express preferred and selected curriculum choices, as a heuristic tool to differentiate theories and methods, as a way of differentiating attitudes and values, as a mechanism to build bridges between related specialties, and as a way of handling the paradoxes in a specialty area such as experimental gerontology. Yet, such applications and usage indicate little appreciation for the entire scope of what Kuhn presented in 1962, and have, in fact, modified it many times over. While we do see predominant theoretical models and favored methodological techniques as well as

privileged application and practice concepts, those who claim there exists a paradigm for gerontology are simply over-reaching or have entirely missed the mark of what paradigm connotes in the philosophy of science. So, we respectfully disagree with the assumption that gerontology has identified itself (by default) with a biomedical paradigm and rather more agree with Ferraro's (2006) assessment that there is a lack of ruling *paradigm,* and, in fact, "the field is only beginning to develop a paradigm" (p. S3).We would argue that our field of gerontology is simply too broad and too wide to experience normal and revolutionary science and any notion of incommensurability between paradigms. What we do have is academic *détente*—an understanding that we go about our business of ageing, respecting the inclusiveness, but in our own ways. But we also claim that a nascent paradigm will not and should not appear, and furthermore, we should not be maneuvering to add any more paradigms to gerontology (Haber 2009) when we never had any to begin with. So we are asking for a cease and desist—an appeal to all, that we step back, and away, from the paradigmatic cliff in gerontology. A paradigm, or set of paradigms, is not possible when we have a primarily atheoretical approach to empirical research in gerontology, a discussion of modernity and postmodernity as it relates to the use of science (see also Sokal and Bricmont 1998), a four-part framework in the *Journals of Gerontology* (biological science, clinical science, behavioral science, and social science), a *Handbook of Theories of Ageing* (Bengtson et al. 2005) with a plurality of "single-aspect" or micro-theories or mid-range theoretical perspectives highlighted (Bengtson et al. 2009), and when there is the call for an integrative model for *social* gerontology—but not the "study of ageing" (Bass 2009). Stating that gerontology (or the study of ageing) is represented by a "multiple paradigm science," or latent, or embryonic, or gerontological imagination, or that it is biomedical, or that it should be empowerment or strengths-based does not help advance our understanding of the scientific structure of gerontology. There is no paradigm and there should not the searching for one in gerontology or the study of ageing: *case closed.* In contrast, we propose that it would be best to proceed by structuring our field as operating in and through *inflection points.*

(4) Finally (as the last stated motivation), the heuristic term of *inflection point* has been used previously and thus there is the precedent for it when used to describe a fundamental shift in a macro-level understanding of the human condition. I am referring to the work of Garreau (2005) and his monumental book, *Radical Evolution: The Promise and Peril of Enhancing Our Minds, Our Bodies—and What it Means to be Human,* in which he examines the following three issues as they relate to technology and bioengineering and their impact on the human condition (p. 6)

- We are riding a curve of exponential change.
- This change is unprecedented in human history.
- It is transforming human nature.

Garreau's (2005) book presents a significant review of and prognosis for the role of four intertwining technologies, known as the GRIN technologies (the genetic, robotic, information, and nano processes) and how these will transform the human experience, including the understanding and meaning of the ageing experience. Here is Garreau (2005), presenting the dynamic of "the curve" (i.e., derivative) as it relates to GRIN technologies,

We are at an inflection point in our history… we have started a wholesale process of aiming our technologies inward. Now our technologies have started to merge with our minds, our memories, our metabolisms, our personalities, our progeny and perhaps our souls (p. 6).

This inflection point will dramatically impact (and to some degree already has) the domain of gerontology and the study of ageing and thus represents the next major transition point for theory, research and practice in the field of ageing for the 21st century.

1.3 A Long Grey Line Revisited and Revised

In an earlier publication titled, *Life in the Long Lane—A Review Essay*, Wright (2008), used the published book by Butler (2008), *The Longevity Revolution: The Benefits and Challenges of Living A Long Life*, as an exemplar for the latest in the "long grey line" of significant contributions in the literature on the topic of senescence. In that paper, Wright (2008) proposed the heuristic phrase a *long grey line* to characterize the extant literature on ageing as essentially a "scatter plot" with the trend line representing a moderate positive correlation, which appeared to culminate with the overarching theme *toward an optimal ageing experience*.

As typical with any scatter plot not every possible example ("point") in the literature is noted as a theoretical point on the graph nor is there any necessary alignment with the trend line as representing the "best fit"; instead, there are varying degrees of correlation with some candidates fitting a low positive correlation in understanding the pattern of graph points, and a few examples even serving as substantial outliers.

As noted by Wright (2008), this "long grey line" has historical roots originating in the mythology of the Greek and Roman era. While some narrative examinations of the ageing experience were characterized as measured, stoical, and grounded in embracing the inevitability of senescence, the trend line representing the flow of works evolves toward a more generous and rewarding theme associated with ageing. The long grey line of literature has become increasingly proscriptive with the presumptive goal of [4.0]: *Optimal Ageing* (including the semantically related phrases of "successful ageing" (Bowling 2007; Dillaway and Byrnes 2009; Inui 2003; Rowe and Khan 1998), "ageing well" (Valliant 2002), "healthy ageing" (Stanner et al. 2009), and a host of related measurable outcomes such as life satisfaction, happiness, and "subjective well-being" (SWB) (see also Krueger 2009). In this book, we embrace the working definition of *optimal ageing* as discussed by Aldwin and Gilmer (2013) such that the optimization of ageing recognizes different ways of ageing well, that people begin with different configurations of ageing vulnerabilities and resources that affect how they age, and that ageing is a process that continually unfolds. But in essence, optimal ageing is defined as a,

> …multidimensional construct that involves avoiding the accelerating agents that promote premature illness and disability, as well as developing protective factors that delay or decelerate the disease and ageing processes to maintain good physical, cognitive, and mental health. (p. 6)

Yet, since the review essay (Wright 2008), we have modified and re-conceptualized the "long grey line" into a series of inflection points that are connected through positive (increasing) derivatives representing the growth in quantity and quality of a particular prevailing trend in gerontological theory, research, and practice (see also Shenk et al. 2001). As noted earlier, the inflection points do not represent paradigm shifts; rather, the threads of previous curvatures interconnect in the sequential shifts in prevailing themes.

References

Achenbaum, A. (1995). *Crossing frontiers: Gerontology emerges as a science*. Cambridge: Cambridge University Press.

Achenbaum, W. A. (2009). A metahistorical perspective on theories of ageing. In V. L. Bengston, D. Gans, N. M. Putney, & M. Silverstein (Eds.), *Handbook of the theories of ageing* (2nd ed., pp. 25–38). New York: Springer.

Adler, F. R. (2012). *Modeling the dynamics of life: Calculus and probability for life scientists* (3rd ed.). Independence: Cengage Learning.

Agamben, G. (2009). *The signature of all things*. New York: Zone Books.

Aldwin, C., & Gilmer, D. (2013). *Health, illness, and optimal ageing: Biological and psychosocial perspectives*. New York: Springer.

Alkema, G., & Alley, D. (2006). Gerontology's future: An integrative model for disciplinary advancement. *Gerontologist, 46*, 574–582.

Alley, D., Putney, N., Rice, M., & Bengtson, V. L. (2010). The increasing use of theory in social gerontology: 1990–2004. *Journal of Gerontology; Social Sciences, 65B*(5), 583–590.

Arendt, H. (2013). *The human condition*. Chicago: University of Chicago Press.

Baltes, P. B., & Nesselroade, J. R. (1984). Paradigm lost and paradigm regained: Critique of dannefer's portrayal of the life span. *American Sociological Review, 49*(6), 841–847.

Bass, S. (2006). Gerontological theory: The search for the holy grail. *Gerontologist, 46*, 139–143.

Bass, S. A. (2009). Toward an integrative theory of social gerontology. In V. Bengtson, M. Silverstein, N. Putney, & D. Gans (Eds.), *Handbook of theories of ageing* (2nd ed., pp. 347–374). New York: Springer.

Bass, S. A., & Ferraro, K. (2000). Gerontology education in transition: Considering disciplinary and paradigmatic evolution. *Gerontologist, 40*(1), 97–106.

Bengtson, V. L., & Schaie, K. W. (1999). *Handbook of theories of ageing*. New York: Springer Publishing Company.

Bengtson, V. L., Rice, C. J., & Johnson, M. L. (1999). Are theories of ageing important? Models and explanations in gerontology at the turn of the century. In V. L. Bengtson & K. W. Schaie (Eds.), *Handbook of the theories of ageing*. New York: Springer.

Bengtson, V. L., Putney, N. M., & Johnson, M. (2005). Ch. 1.2. Are theories of ageing necessary? In M. Johnson, V. L. Bengtson, P. Coleman, & T. Kirkwood, (Eds.), *The Cambridge handbook of age and ageing*. Cambridge: Cambridge University Press.
Bengtson, V. L., Gans, D., Putney, N., & Silverstein, M. (2009). *Handbook of theories of ageing*. New York: Springer Publishing.
Bhopal, R. (1999). Paradigms in epidemiology textbooks: In the footsteps of Thomas Kuhn. *American Journal of Public Health, 89*(8), 1162–1165.
Biggs, S., Lowenstein, A., & Hendricks, J. (2003). The need for theory in gerontology. In S. Biggs, A. Lowenstein, & J. Hendricks (Eds.), *The need for theory: Critical approaches to social gerontology* (pp. 1–14). New York: Baywood.
Blackmore, S. (2004). *Consciousness: An introduction*. New York: Oxford University Press.
Boghossian, P. (2006). *Fear of knowledge: Against relativism and constructivism*. New York: Oxford University Press.
Bowling, A. (2007). Aspirations for older age in the 21s[t] century: What is successful ageing? *International Journal of Human Development, 64*(3), 263–297.
Brient, E. (2001). From vita contemplativa to vita activa: Modern instrumentalization of theory and the problem of measure. *International Journal of Philosophical Studies, 9*, 19–40.
Brockman, J. (1995). *The third culture: Beyond the scientific revolution*. New York: Simon & Schuster.
Butler, R. (2008). *The longevity revolution: The benefits and challenges of living a long life*. New York: Public Affairs.
Caneva, K. (2000). Possible Kuhns in the history of science: Anomalies of incommensurable paradigms. *Studies in History and Philosophy of Science, 31*(1), 87–124.
Carpi, M., Salvioli, S., Monti, D., Caruso, C., Candore, G., & Vasto, S. (2008). Human longevity within an evolutionary perspective: The peculiar paradigm of a post-reproductive genetics. *Experimental Gerontology, 43*, 53–60.
Carvalho, J. (2006). Overview of the structure of a scientific worldview. *Zygon, 41*(1), 113–124.
Chapin, R., & Cox, E. O. (2001). Changing the paradigm: Strengths-based and empowerment-oriented social work with frail elders. *Journal of Gerontological Social Work, 36*(3/4), 165–179.
Charness, N. (2004). Preface. In D. C. Brudick, & S. Kwon. (Eds.), *Gerotechnology: Research and practice in technology and ageing* (pp. xxv). New York: Springer.
Cole, T. R. (1992). *The journey of life: A cultural history of ageing in America*. New York: Cambridge University Press.
Cole, T. R., Ray, R., & Kastenbaum, R. (2010). *A guide to humanistic studies in ageing*. Baltimore: The Johns Hopkins University Press.
Conant, J., & Haugeland, J. (2000). *The road since structure: Philosophical essays, 1970–1993 with an autobiographical interview*. Chicago, IL: University of Chicago Press.
Costa, G. D. N. (Trans.). (2005). *Seneca: On the shortness of life*. New York: Penguin Books. (Original work published 56 A. D.).
Critser, G. (2010). *Eternity soup: Inside the quest to end ageing*. New York: Harmony Books.
Cutler, S. (2005). Ageism and technology. *Generations, 23*(3), 67–72.
Cutler, S. (2006). Technological change and ageing. In R. Binstock & L. George (Eds.), *Handbook of ageing and the social sciences* (6th ed., pp. 257–276). San Diego: Academic Press.
Dannefer, D., & Daub, A. (2009). Extending the interrogation: Life span, life course, and the constitution of human ageing. *Advances in Life Course Research, 14*, 15–27.
Dawkins, R. (2009). *The greatest show on earth: the evidence for evolution*. New York: Free Press.
Diewald, M., & Mayer, K. U. (2009). The sociology of the life course and life span psychology: Integrated paradigm or complementing pathways? *Advances in Life Course Research, 14*, 5–14.

Dillaway, H., & Byrnes, M. (2009). Reconsidering successful ageing: A call for renewed and expanded academic critiques and conceptualizations. *Journal of Applied Gerontology, 28*(6), 702–722.

Ferrario, C. G., Freeman, F. J., Nellet, G., & Scheel, J. (2008). Changing nursing student's attitudes about ageing: An argument for the successful ageing paradigm. *Educational Gerontology, 34*(1), 51–66.

Ferraro, K. (2006). Imagining the disciplinary advancement of gerontology: Whither the tipping point? *The Gerontologist, 46*, 571–573.

Garreau, J. (2005). *Radical evolution: The promise and peril of enhancing our minds, our bodies—and What It means to be human*. New York: Broadway (Random House).

Gay, V. (2010). *Progress and values in the humanities: comparing culture and science*. New York: Columbia University Press.

Gigerenzer, G. (2008). *Rationality for mortals: How people cope with uncertainty*. New York: Oxford University Press.

Gigerenzer, G., Czerlinski, J., & Martignon, L. (2002). How good are fast and frugal heuristics? In T. Gilovich, D. Griggin, & D. Kahneman (Eds.), *Heuristics and biases: The psychology of intuitive judgment* (pp. 559–581). New York: Cambridge University Press.

Gill, C. (2013). *Marcus Aurelius: Meditations*. Oxford: Oxford University Press.

Groner, R., Groner, M., & Bischof, W. F. (Eds.). (1983). *Methods of heuristics*. Hillsdale: Lawrence Erlbaum Associates, Publishers.

Haber, D. (2009). Gerontology: Adding an empowerment paradigm. *Journal of Applied Gerontology, 28*(3), 283–297.

Hendricks, J., & Achenbaum, W. A. (1999). Historical development of theories of ageing. In V. L. Bengtson & K. W. Schaie (Eds.), *Handbook of theories of ageing* (pp. 21–39). New York: Springer Publishing.

Hung, E. H. (2001). Kuhnian paradigms as representational spaces: New perspectives on the problems of incommensurability, scientific explanation, and physical necessity. *Internal Studies in the Philosophy of Science, 15*(3), 275–292.

Inui, T. S. (2003). The need for an integrated biopsychological approach to research on successful ageing. *Annals of Internal Medicine, 139*, 391–394.

Kagan, J. (2009). *The three cultures: Natural sciences, social sciences, and the humanities in the 21st century*. New York: Cambridge University Press.

Katz, S. (1996). *Disciplining old age: The formation of gerontological knowledge*. Charlottesville: The University Press of Virginia.

Katz, J. E. (Ed.). (2003).*Machines that become us: The social context of interpersonal communication technologies*. New Brunswick: Transaction Publishers.

Kaye, L. W., Butler, S. S., & Webster, N. M. (2003). Toward a productive ageing paradigm for geriatric practice. *Ageing International, 28*(2), 200–213.

Krueger, A. B. (2009). *Measuring the subjective well-being of nations: National accounts of time use and well-being*. Chicago: The University of Chicago Press.

Kuhn, T. S. (1970). *The structure of scientific revolutions*. Chicago: University of Chicago Press.

Kuhn, T. S. (1977). *the essential tension: selected studies in scientific Tradition and change*. Chicago: University of Chicago Press.

Kuhn, T. S. (2000). *The road since structure. Philosophical essays 1970–1993*. Chicago: University of Chicago Press.

Lakatos, I. (1970). Falsification and the methodology of scientific research programmes. In I. Lakatos & A. Musgrave (Eds.), *Criticism and the growth of knowledge*. New York: Cambridge University Press.

Laudan, L. (1984). *Science and values*. Berkeley: University of California Press.

Lehrer, J. (2009). *How we decide*. Boston: Houghton Mifflin Harcourt.

Marsh, B., Todd, P. M., & Gigerenzer, G. (2004). Cognitive heuristics: Reasoning the fast and frugal way. In J. Leighton & R. Sternberg (Eds.), *The nature of reasoning* (pp. 273–287). New York: Cambridge University Press.

Mayo, D. (1996). Ducks, rabbits, and normal science: Recasting the kuhn's-eye view of popper's demarcation of science. *The British Journal for the Philosophy of Science, 47*(2), 271–290.

Mayr, E. (1994). The advance of science and scientific revolutions. *Journal of the History of Behavioral Sciences, 30*, 328–334.

O'Donohue, W. (1992). Is gerontology a branch of astrology? The role of advanced age in scientific explanation. *New Ideas in Psychology, 10*(3), 321–329.

O'Donohue, W. (1993). The spell of Kuhn on psychology: An exegetical elixir. *Philosophical Psychology, 6*(3), 267–288.

Popper, K. (1963). *Conjectures and refutations*. London: Routledge & Kegan Paul.

Powell, J. L. (2009). Social theory, and health and welfare professionals: A Foucauldian, "toolkit". *Journal of Applied Gerontology, 28*(6), 669–682.

Radder, H. (1997). Philosophy and history of science: Beyond the Kuhnian paradigm. *Studies in History and Philosophy of Science, 28*(4), 633–655.

Ramachandran, V. S. (2004). *A brief Tour of human consciousness*. New York: PI Press.

Read, C. Y., Green, R. C., & Smyer, M. A. (Eds.). (2008). *Ageing, biotechnology, and the future*. Baltimore: The Johns Hopkins University Press.

Rickman, H. (2004). *The riddle of the sphinx: Interpreting the human world.* Cranbury: Associated University Presses.

Roberts, M. J. (2004). Heuristics and reasoning I: Making deduction simple. In J. Leighton & R. Sternberg (Eds.), *The nature of reasoning* (pp. 234–272). New York: Cambridge University Press.

Rowe, J. W., & Kahn, R. L. (1998). *Successful ageing*. New York: Pantheon Books.

Scheffer, M. (2009). *Critical transitions in nature and society*. Princeton: Princeton University Press.

Schmidt, L. K. (2006). *Understanding hermeneutics*. Stocksfield: Acumen.

Settersten, R. (2006). Ageing and the life course. In R. Binstock, & L. George (Eds.), *Handbook of ageing and the social sciences* (pp. 3–20). New York: Academic Press.

Settersten, R. A. (2009). It takes two to tango: The (un)easy dance between life-course sociology and life-span psychology. *Advances in Life Course Research, 14*, 74–81.

Shapin, S. (2010). *Never pure: Historical studies of people as if it was produced by people with bodies, situated in time, space, culture, and society, and struggling for credibility and authority*. Baltimore: The Johns Hopkins University Press.

Shenk, D.,Rowles, G.,Peacock, J. R.,Mitchell, J.,Fisher, B. J.,Moore, K. S., & Hare, L. (2001). Teaching research in gerontology: toward a cumulative model. *Educational Gerontology, (27)*7, 537–556.

Sherraden, M., Morrow-Howell, N., Hinterlong, J., & Rozario, P. (2001). Productive ageing: Theoretical choices and directions. In N. Morrow-Howell, J. Hinterlong, & M. Sherraden (Eds.), *Productive ageing: Concerns and challenges* (pp. 260–284). Baltimore: The Johns Hopkins University Press.

Slingerland, E. (2008). *What science offers the humanities: Integrating body and culture*. New York: Cambridge University Press.

Snow, C. P. (1964). *The two cultures and a second look: An expanded version of the two cultures and the scientific revolution*. New York: Cambridge University Press (Canto Edition).

Sokal, A., & Bricmont, J. (1998). *Fashionable nonsense: Postmodern intellectuals' abuse of science*. New York: Picador.

Sophocles (2005). *Oedipus at Colonus*. (E. Grennan & M. R. Kitzinger, Trans.). New York: Oxford University Press. (Original work published 401 B.C.).

Stanner, S., Thompson, R., & Buttriss, J. L. (2009). *Healthy ageing: The role of nutrition and lifestyle*. Oxford: Wiley-Blackwell.

Suppe, F. (1977). *The structure of scientific theories*. Urbana: University of Illinois Press.

Tauber, A. I. (2009). *Science and the quest for meaning*. Waco: Baylor University Press.

Valliant, G. (2002). *Ageing well: Surprising guideposts to a happier life from the landmark harvard study of adult development*. Boston: Little Brown.

Von Dietze, E. (2001). *Paradigms explained: Rethinking Thomas Kuhn's philosophy of science*. Westport: Praeger.

Weaver, J. W. (1999). Gerontology education: A new paradigm for the 21st century. *Educational Gerontology, 25*, 479–490.

Weaver, K., & Olson, J. (2006). Understanding paradigms used for nursing research. *Journal of Advanced Nursing, 53*(4), 459–469.

Weisstein, E. W. (2009). Inflection point. *From MathWorld—A Wolfram Web Resource*. Retrieved from http://mathworld.wolfram.com/InflectionPoint.html.

Wilmoth, J., & Ferraro, K. (2007). The fountain of gerontological discovery. In J. Wilmoth & K. Ferraro (Eds.), *Gerontology: Perspectives and issues* (3rd ed., pp. 3–12). New York: Springer Publishing.

Wilson, E. O. (1998). *Consilience*. New York: Alfred A. Knopf.

Wimsatt, W. C. (2007). *Re-Engineering philosophy for limited beings: Piecewise approximations to reality*. Cambridge: Cambridge University Press.

Wright, S. D. (2008). Life in the long lane—a review essay on the longevity revolution: The benefits and challenges of living a long life by Robert N. Butler. *Journal of the American Heart Association*, *2*(3/4), 298–313.

Chapter 2
The Definition and Delineation of Each Inflection Point

Abstract And so we postulate that the call to reinstate the themes of "fate and mutability, mortality and finitude, suffering and wisdom" (see Cole 1992, p. 243) are certainly noble ideals; nevertheless, they have been swept aside by the rising tide of a postmodern culture that has not only embraced the ever-expanding sphere of the "ageing industry" (Estes 1979, 1993) but has taken the scientific management of ageing and morphed it into many macro-level extensions of a "scientific-industrial" complex emerging out of the 1950s.There may be a "new ageing enterprise" (Moody 2004/2005, 2008) on the rise, but we argue that there has not been any relinquishment of the hegemony found with the "positive" pole of the duality (i.e., the striving toward an optimal ageing) and instead, ironically, there is the emerging value-laden zeitgeist in gerontology that seems to embrace only the *way forward*—exponentially—without much regard for premodern, modern or postmodern *values of ageing* at all.

Keywords Ageing as a reflection · Ageing as a problem · Ageing as a challenge · Ageing as a reward · Ageing as an artifact · Ageing demographics · Ageing population · Biomedical technology · Blue zones · Bioengineering · Human longevity · Senescence · Shortgevity · Social disparities

2.1 [1.0]: Philosophy of Ageing (Ageing as a *Reflection*)

Wright (2008) proposed that the long grey trend line extended through such works as Sophocles' *Oedipus at Colonus,* Marcus Aurelius' *Meditations*, was later synthesized in Tim Parkin's contemporary book, *Old Age in the Roman World: A Cultural and Social History*, and with Moog and Schäfer's article, "Joannes Stobaios, 'On Old Age': An Important Source for the History of Gerontology" which also examines Cicero's well-known text "On Old Age" (*Cato maior de senectute*). Re-conceptualized for our new approach of *inflection points*, this was the first positive derivative [1.0] for the curvature *Philosophy of Ageing*. We

K.F. Felsted and S.D. Wright, *Toward Post Ageing*,
Healthy Ageing and Longevity 1, DOI 10.1007/978-3-319-09051-1_2

propose that Arthur Schopenhauer (1788–1860) represents an exemplar contributor of the *Philosophy of Ageing*, and perhaps its zenith as well (Edman 1928; Hannan 2009; Magee 1997).We submit that the chapter, "The Ages of Life," in Schopenhauer's book (2008) *The Wisdom of Life and Counsels and Maxims* (see excerpt following) is an indication of Schopenhauer's attempt to answer the "riddle of the world" (Hannan 2009) in terms of the human condition,

> From the point of view we have been taking up until now, life may be compared to a piece of embroidery, of which, during the first half of his time, a man gets a sight of the right side, and during the second half, of the wrong. The wrong side is not so pretty as the right, but it is more instructive; it shows the way in which the threads have been worked together (p. 123).

This philosophical drive to solve the "riddle of the world" sounds like a continuation of the ancient riddle of the sphinx that confronted Oedipus with a supposed mystery along the life course: *What walks on four legs in the morning, two legs at noon, and three legs in the evening?* Of course, Oedipus solved the riddle, answering that it was man that crawls on all fours in infancy, walks upright on two legs in adulthood, and uses a cane as a third leg in old age. Hannan (2009) also offers an interesting insight that relates to our exposition here in this book,

> Schopenhauer was a transitional thinker, bridging the gap between nineteenth-century and twentieth-century paradigms. It is typical of such transitional thinkers that are officially working within a framework that they are also (half-consciously) pushing toward a new epistemology in which both science and metaphysics, seamlessly blending into each other, both depend and do not depend on experience (p. 15).

Schopenhauer is the exemplar of the tradition of the *Philosophy of Ageing*, yet his influence and that of others before him (e.g., Marcus Aurelius, Seneca) still resonate as influential threads for scholars (e.g., Freud, Jung, Levinson) into the next inflection point [2.0] and beyond. It does appear that we have skimmed over many centuries of literature from the works of Sophocles, Seneca, and Marcus Aurelius to Schopenhauer, but we are attempting to stay engaged with the primary purpose of this book in the examination of inflection points and the ageing experience from a historical viewpoint. Nevertheless, we will privilege the following works to serve as supplementary texts for those professionals with an interest in the study of ageing who prefer to use the "long view" perspective and would then be well advised to consider for further reading to cover the significant transitions from the *Philosophy of Ageing*, [1.0] or ageing as a *reflection*, to the *Bio-medical Diseases of Ageing*, [2.0] or ageing as a *problem*:

From Dawn to Decadence: 1500 *to present* (500 *years of Western Cultural Life*) by Barzun (2000); *The Dream of Reason; A History of Philosophy from the Greeks to the Renaissance* by Gottlieb (2002); *A Secular Age* by Taylor (2007); *History of the Twentieth Century* by Gilbert (2001); *The Problem of the Soul* by Flanagan (2002); *The Crooked Timber of Humanity* by Berlin (1990), *Flesh in the Age of Reason: The Modern Foundations of Body and Soul* by Porter (2003), and *The Age of Wonder: How the Romantic Generation Discovered the Beauty and Terror of Science* by Holmes (2009; also recommended is the review of this book by Freeman Dyson in *New York Review of Books*, Aug. 19, 2009). We would place the modern publication, *The Oxford Book of Ageing: Reflections on the Journey of Life*, edited by Cole and Winkler (1994), the publication *Journal of Ageing, Humanities, and the Arts* (JAHA); the book by Quinodoz (2010), *Growing Old: A Journey of Self-Discovery*; Charney's book (2009) *Wrinkled in Time: Ageing Shakespeare*; and *A Guide to Humanistic Studies in Ageing: What Does It Mean to Grow Old?* (Cole et al. 2010).

2.2 [2.0]: The Bio-Medical Diseases of Ageing (Ageing as a *Problem*)

The second positive derivative [2.0], the Bio-medical Diseases of Ageing (or ageing as a *problem*) is identified approximately with the beginning of the 20th century with the advent of both specialties investigating the phenomenon of ageing as a problem to be addressed scientifically: gerontology and geriatrics (Achenbaum 2001). Exemplars are represented by Sanford Bennett Dodd *Old Age: Its Cause and Prevention*, and readers should note the related stories of reversing ageing by Mircea Eliade, *Youth Without Youth,* and F. Scott Fitzgerald, *The Curious Case of Benjamin Button* (see Alexander 2009), both of which were recently made into movies, respectively by Francis Ford Coppola 2007, and David Fincher 2008. Then came Hall's (1922) *Senescence: The Last Half of Life* and another book, titled *Old Age: The Major Involution: The Physiology and Pathology of the Ageing Process*, by Alfred Scott Warthin (1930). And in the 1930s, there was Carl Jung's (1933) insightful chapter, "The Stages of Life" in *Modern Man In Search of Soul*, which we believe carries on threads from the Philosophy of Ageing [1.0] curvature. Moving upward along the positive curvature of [2.0], Ageing, *The Biology of Senescence,* was written by Comfort (1964) and soon after came the deeper reflections of de Beauvoir (1972) in her book, *The Coming of Age.* We then move upward to *Ageing and Mental Health: Positive Psychosocial Approaches* by Butler and Lewis (1973). We could explore the textured dimensions of ageing captured in *The Psychology of Adult Development and Ageing* edited by Eisdorfer and Powell Lawton (1973)and then continue on to another hallmark publication (and Pulitzer Prize winning book) by Butler (1975), *Why Survive? Being Old in America.* And, in the following year, *A Good Age* by Comfort (1976).

And it is here, in the time frame of the late 1970s and early 1980s that we propose that the third inflection point is initiated: [3.0] Demographics of Ageing (ageing as a *challenge*). Yet the active threads of [2.0] curvature are still present, but not as dramatically positive compared to the next derivative, and strongly identified in contemporary publications such as *Hazzard's Geriatric Medicine & Gerontology, Sixth Edition: Principles of Geriatric Medicine & Gerontology* (Halter et al. 2009). As Bass (2007) has noted, "Gerontology in the early 1980s was very much focused on the frailty, dependence, and decline in later life" (p. 135), and we will further propose while it was the prevailing trend, it would soon be dominated by a more macro-level perspective that would take the "ageing as problem" theme and transform it into "ageing as a challenge" due to demographic transitions already underway in developed countries—and with the looming challenge of ageing baby boomers ahead.

2.3 [3.0] Demographics of Ageing (Ageing as a *Challenge*)

This change in direction along the curvature is clearly indicated by exemplars of several publications such as the edited book by Pifer and Bronte (1986b), *Our Ageing Society: Paradox and Promise* (see also Pifer and Bronte 1986a). As proposed by our heuristic model, there are also several publications that carry over the threads from previous inflection points such as Cole's (1992). *The Journey of Life: A Cultural History of Ageing in America* which we consider more of meta-theoretical and historiography of both [1.0] and [2.0] curvatures.The publication, *The New Ageing: Politics and Change in America* by Torres-Gil (1992) clearly falls along the direction of the [3.0] inflection point. We consider Hayflick's (1994) *How and Why We Age* as a continuing thread from the [2.0] curvature, while Amery's (1994) publication, *On Ageing: Revolt and Resignation,* carried the philosophical gravity of the [1.0] curvature with strong narrative reflecting the philosophy of the ageing process. Then there was Posner's (1995) *Ageing and Old Age* which strongly influenced the [3.0] positive derivative.We then capture Roszak's (1998). *America the Wise: the Longevity Revolution and the True Wealth of Nations*, later expanded and revised to be published again in 2001 under the title of *Longevity Revolution: As Boomers Become Elders* (Roszak 2001), as a part of the [3.0] curvature, along with Peterson's (1999) less than optimistic outlook about ageing as a problem, *Gray Dawn: How the Coming Age Wave Will Transform America and the World*, but then the counterweight publication of *Age Power: How the 21st Century Will Be Ruled by the New Old* by Dychtwald (1999). The publication *The Quest for Immortality: Science at the Frontiers of Ageing* by Olshansky and Carnes (2001) represents a cross-weave of threads for [2.0] and [3.0] curvatures and offers a cautious indicator into the curvature of [4.0]. Friedan's (1993) *The Fountain of Age* served to break new ground between [3.0] and the next inflection point to follow, [4.0]: Optimal Ageing. Sheehy's (1996) *New Passages: Mapping Your Life Across Time*, continues the trend of Betty Freidan's work to become an influence on the [4.0] curvature toward optimal ageing.

But perhaps the exemplar for this [3.0] inflection point and representation of an ongoing thread for the previous prevailing theme was the publication, *International Handbook of Population Ageing* (Uhlenberg 2009) which offered thirty-four chapters on various topics ranging from migration patterns and economic issues, to the interconnection with health care issues. Of all those chapters, the one chapter that we see representing a "bridge" into inflection point [5.0]: Post Ageing was authored by Olshansky and Carnes (2009), *The Future of Human Longevity*. We believe this is a bridge publication not so much for any "pro" post ageing stance they might have taken (which they did not); on the contrary, it is because they represented that rare breed of scholar that would look beyond their limited silo of research emphasis (and prevailing view of [3.0]) and critically examine the implications and consequences of technologies for human longevity. In that chapter by Olshansky and Carnes (2009), they present a very convincing and explicit profile for "pathways to longer life" and propose that there are three camps with differing perspectives and viewpoints about the prospect for human longevity. The three groups are: *the futurists, the optimists*, and *the realists*, and we will further discuss them in the next sections.

Relevant to the discussion of [3.0], however, Olshansky and Carnes (2009) believe it is the first group of researchers and writers, known as the *futurists*, who are invested in "yet-to-be developed advances in biomedical technology and the anticipated emergence of nanotechnology are going to radically transform the landscape of human ageing and longevity" (p. 731).It should be pointed out that Olshansky and Carnes (2009), fitting in the [3.0] curvature, do not find any compelling evidence for either the *futurists* or the *optimists* to gain traction for dramatically changing the limits of human longevity beyond the 88 years for women and 82 years for men, unless there were a technological breakthrough "capable of slowing the rate of biological ageing" and that the breakthrough could also be "broadly disseminated" (p. 732). Although we are assertively presenting a case for the next inflection point and we have a (now self-disclosed) degree of affinity with the "futurist" camp (although we do find the label a bit awkward and loaded with metaphysical trappings), we also find the "realist" label of Olshansky and Carnes (and their preferred stance) to be a sobering and needed counterweight to the overreach of several futurists involved in "post ageing" speculations (see also Bongaarts 2009). Nevertheless, it is our assertion that they have underestimated the potential impact for technologies to alter the current prevailing viewpoint from [4.0] Optimal Ageing to a [5.0] Post Ageing curvature. We also submit that they have over-extrapolated the lack of successes in the historical track record of human endeavors in trying to extend the life span. In other words, we do not think that past is prologue—especially in the case of technological advancements affecting the ageing process. Finally, we believe they have too narrowly defined the role of futurists as succumbing to the allure of immortality as the main motivation (or preoccupation) for who would study—*and advance*—the intersect of technologies in the domain of ageing. Yet, we do credit Olshansky and Carnes (2009) in identifying a weakness in the realist's argument that is, ironically, related to the possible and potential advancement in bio-medical technologies exceeding the limits of human longevity. Our point is that Olshansky and Carnes (2009) (and also Bongaarts 2009) at least concede that going beyond these limits is possible, without seeing any near-term advancements to create this change on the visible horizon. A final point: we are in complete agreement with them that any developments and advancements in extending human longevity due to breakthrough technologies would have to be *broadly disseminated* to avoid the specter that only a select few—or an elite group—couldbenefit from such advancements.

The latest publications that represent the continuation of [3.0] would be: (1) the report hosted by the U.S. Census Bureau and National Institute of Ageing titled, *An Ageing World: 2008* (Kinsella and He 2009).This report indicated that although the world's population is ageing, children still outnumber older people as of 2008. However, projections indicate, that in fewer than 10 years, *older people will outnumber children* for the first time in history; (2) the two-volume publication edited by Hudson (2009) titled, *Boomer Bust? Economic and Political Issues of the Graying Society* (Volume 1: Perspectives on the Boomers; Volume 2: The Boomers and Their Future). Hudson (2009) presented an impressive array of authors primarily in the domains of economics, political science, and finance to *challenge* the notion that ageing baby boom cohort is a recipe for disaster; (3) the working paper by Preston and Ho (2009), "Low Life Expectancy in the United States: Is the Health Care System at Fault?" and, (4) research supported by the MacArthur Foundation, "Ageing in America in the Twenty-First Century: Demographics Forecasts from the MacArthur Foundation Research Network on an Ageing Society" by Olshansky et al. (2009) who propose that both the U.S. Social Security Administration and U.S. Census Bureau may have *underestimated* the rise in life expectancy for both men and women in the U.S. Olshansky et al. (2009) further indicated that the risk of death in the coming decades will be reduced by *accelerated advances in biomedical technology* that delay the onset and progression of major fatal diseases or that slow the ageing process.

2.4 [4.0]: Optimal Ageing (Ageing as a *Reward*)

> The Longevity Dividend doesn't suggest that we live longer; instead it calls for living better. The idea is that if we use science to increase healthspan, not lifespan. In other words, tomorrow's 50-year-old would have the health profile of a 43-year-old.
> ~ *Gray is the New Gold: State of the Science in Two Thousand Nine* (2009). [Optimism in Ageing Research]. Kronos Longevity Research Institute (KLRI) (p. 4).

The next inflection point, and what we propose is the current prevailing theme in gerontology, is posited to have taken place in the mid- to late 1990s with the full positive derivative effect expressed with the turn of the century (the year 2000). The following represent exemplars of this change in direction for the curvature: *The Creative Age: Awakening Human Potential In The Second Half Of Life* (Cohen 2001); *Productive Ageing: Concepts and Challenges* (Morrow-Howell et al 2001); *Challenges of the Third Age: Meaning and Purpose in Later Life* (Weiss and Bass 2002); Valliant (2002) and his work, *Ageing Well: Surprising Guideposts to a Happier Life*; and *Positive Ageing* (Hill 2005). As stated in the proposal of inflection points there are threads of previous prevailing themes that carry over into the subsequent curvatures, and the book *Challenges of an Ageing Society: Ethical Dilemmas, Political Issues* edited by Pruchno and Smyer (2007) represents such an exemplar. We approach the final exemplars of [4.0] with Nuland's (2007) *The Art of Ageing: A Doctor's Prescription for Well-being,* and Goldsmith's (2008). *The Long Baby Boom: An Optimistic Vision for a Graying*

Generation, and then Butler's (2008) book, *The Longevity Revolution.* We propose that Robert Butler's book is the literary capstone work for indicating the incremental works on the experience of ageing as essentially an optimistic endeavor and the triumphal and prevailing theme (optimal ageing) for all of gerontology.

In other words, according to some, we have reached the point whereby we can begin to reap the benefits of the so-called "longevity dividend" (Kronos Longevity Research Institute [KLRI] 2009).However, Butler (2008) admitted that there is much work to be done and there were significant threats to sustaining an increase in longevity, notably in those geographic areas that are characterized by "short-gevity" (International Longevity Center Global Alliance 2009). Nevertheless, Butler was cautiously optimistic that the future is now if we are to reap the rewards of increased longevity, and that there is an attitude of making good use of the tools that we have, and hope to have, to enjoy "the triumphant prolongation of life." So, although the longevity revolution has both benefits and challenges, the overarching tone is progressive and the faith in the scientific enterprise's ability to address the challenges of increasing longevity is unwavering. For example, Butler (2008) noted in the preface of his book that,

> Scientific advancements should and will add vigor and health throughout life, and not just at its end. The ageing population increasingly consists of active, vigorous, robust people. We must not take them for granted, but the trend can continue and it should be celebrated. Above all, I hope that this book will convince people that our increased longevity constitutes a supreme achievement (p. vx).

More recently, Robine et al. (2013), as editors of *Healthy Longevity, A Global Approach* (Volume 33 of the *Annual Review of Gerontology and Geriatrics*) explore healthy longevity as a theoretical concept. We do not go so far as to claim a teleological argument or grand narrative to be found within the exemplars already, but we are in agreement with Cole (1992) that the "long-term transition from the existential to scientific tonalities" in our understanding of the ageing experience has led us to this point on the trend line. Cole elaborates,

> Since the mid-nineteenth century, Americans have come to view ageing not as a fated aspect of our individual and social existence, but as one of life's problems to be solved through willpower, aided by science, technology, and expertise (pp. xxii—xxiii).

Having said that, Cole (1992) was not sure that the assumed outcome of all the supposed scientific activity was going to necessarily be a positive gain for humanity. Cole was skeptical about "successful ageing" models serving as the end game to such scientific endeavors as they tend toward the too idealistic while negating the harsh realities of decline and death. Cole believed that the authority of the scientific management model "with its drive to maximize health and organic functioning" had stripped away existential meaning that addresses the paradoxical nature of ageing and had instead replaced it with a "relentless hostility to physical decline and its tendency to regard health as a form of secular salvation" (p. 239). In other words, the scientific management of ageing has come at a high spiritual and ethical price. Cole (1992) believed that the emergence of a duality, a dichotomous treatment of the ageing experience, had become the guiding paradigm in the field of ageing,

> Rooted in the drive for unlimited individual accumulation of health and wealth, this dualism has hindered our culture's ability to sustain morally compelling social practices and existentially vital ideals of ageing (Cole 1992, p. 230).

And from this duality, the positive pole would facilitate the perspective of optimal ageing: "Old people are (or should be) healthy, sexually active, engaged, productive, and self-reliant" (p. 229).This perspective is also represented in the emergent domain of positive psychology as it intersects with ageing (Hill 2005) as well as with the call to understand and promote "blue zones" as viable geographic and social areas that encourage health lifestyles leading to a longer life expectancies (Buettner 2008).

And yet, Cole believed that the postmodern cultural era (see also Butler) able to reflect a deepening existential awareness of the ageing experience and thus seen as much more than a "problem to be solved." Indeed, Cole believed that the "modern quest for a rational, healthy, and orderly life course has reached a limit—or at least a turning point." Cole called upon the possibility of the postmodern self to "cultivate the existential nourishment" (perhaps through the arts as example) along the life course. But Cole's scholarly work was first published in 1992, and given that a substantial amount of time has since passed, it all begs the question to ask—and then determine—if his hoped for potential has actually been initiated, much less realized, as we approach the year 2015, some twenty two years later (see also Cole et al. 2010).

2.5 Forecasting a Significant Change in the Present Curvature

And so we offer a synopsis at this juncture of the book in order to provisionally measure the significant and substantial attainment of the hoped for emergence of "vital postmodern ideals of ageing" that perhaps relates to larger rubric of "humanistic gerontology" (Cole et al. 2000; Cole and Sierpina 2007). In other words, although we are posing the question, we will nevertheless take the tactical move in this book and advance our diagnosis, but we will then propose an entirely *different* prognosis, than what Cole and fellow supporters had hoped for, of what lies ahead. At this juncture, we also want to be clear about our stance on the premise and goals of a *humanistic gerontology*: We are in full support of this approach for the understanding of the ageing experience both personally and professionally. As faculty members in a gerontology program, we embrace the significance of interdisciplinary approach for the study of ageing and weave that structure and attitude into our curriculum content so that a full spectrum of conceptual models, theories, and methodologies are presented. This spectrum of perspectives ranges from the molecular to the molar—from the study of telomeres to the examination of macro-level policies on ageing at the national and global level.

And so to put it most diplomatically, we are *not* convinced that such a movement (or any actuality) for any "postmodern ideal of ageing" has taken hold and gained traction in our culture. While we concede that *optimal ageing* is our prevailing theme (notice we did not say "paradigm") in gerontology, and that there are a few exceptions representing the spirit of the ideal to be found with the intersect of ageing baby boomers and civic engagement (e.g., the work carried out by the Civic Ventures organization and Encore) we submit that the return to "meaning" (see Krause 2009), in large part a balanced return to the grand humanistic tradition of the ageing experience, has been left to fend for itself with well-intentioned advocates and devotees (to which Cole and Sierpina 2007, seem to agree as they identify this group as an "important minority" p. 252) in the few remaining and somewhat secluded islands of publications such as the emergence of the *Handbook of the Humanities and Ageing* (Cole et al. 2000), *A Guide to Humanistic Studies in Ageing: What Does it Mean to Grow Old?* (Cole et al. 2010), and the journal *Journal of Ageing, Humanities, and the Arts (JAHA).* We entirely support these publications and outlets, but at the same time we are confident that the perspective of "humanistic gerontology" will not be able to withstand the emergence and forthcoming predominance of new and more powerful forces in scientific endeavors (which is the proposed [5.0] inflection point underway) resulting from the *convergence* of bioengineering and technology in gerontology.

And so we postulate that the call to reinstate the themes of "fate and mutability, mortality and finitude, suffering and wisdom" (see Cole 1992, p. 243) are certainly noble ideals; nevertheless, they have been swept aside by the rising tide of a postmodern culture that has not only embraced the ever-expanding sphere of the "ageing industry" (Estes 1979, 1993) but has taken the scientific management of ageing and morphed it into many macro-level extensions of a "scientific-industrial" complex emerging out of the 1950s. There may be a "new ageing enterprise" (Moody, 2004/2005, 2008) on the rise, but we argue that there has not been any relinquishment of the hegemony found with the "positive" pole of the duality (i.e., the striving toward an optimal ageing) and instead, ironically, there is the emerging value-laden zeitgeist in gerontology that seems to embrace only the *way forward*—exponentially—without much regard for premodern, modern or postmodern *values of ageing* at all.

In fact the postmodern era has splintered itself into a myriad of conditions with the prefix "post" to be found almost connected to everything traditionally studied and practiced (e.g., post-colonial, post-structuralist, postdigital, postbiological, postAmerican, and posthuman). In fact, some have proposed that we have already moved beyond postmodernism (if it ever existed; see Matthewman and Hoey 2006) and into a "digimodernism" that reflects more of the digital and technological culture (Kirby 2009). This grammatical and "paradigmatic" shift in tone and temporal development signals that some kind of conceptual train (i.e., epistemological, theoretical, methodological, ontological) has already left the academic station. Although some may wish for us to consider "gerontology's future" by the privileging of three main disciplines: *biology, psychology*, and *sociology* into an "integrative model" and perhaps even embrace gerontology's entry into the disciplinary status due to identified accomplishments thus far (Alkema and Alley 2006), others such as Ferraro (2006) are not so sure that the critical mass is there yet. In either case, whether one is "pro-discipline" and advocates as though "it" has arrived, or if rather one believes like Ferraro (2006) that such a tipping point is still "several cohorts away" from achieving the laurel wreath representing a bona fide academic discipline, or perhaps if one believes that the *disciplinary evolution* will never happen, it is a major limitation to neglect to recognize the *bio-technological* in the tenets of a *gerontological imagination* in addressing the ageing experience as we begin to experience the next inflection point of Post Ageing [5.0].

And so despite the calls for a new focus in the field of ageing to balance the control of the natural sciences (Cole and Sierpina 2007) such as Haber's (2009) suggestion of an "Empowerment Paradigm" for and about ageing boomers, we contend that this simply represents a continuation, an extension of the prevailing *optimal ageing* curvature [4.0] or the positive pole in Cole's duality, that has already had its peak opportunity.

In other words, the optimal ageing theme has been the predominant pathway and compass within the gerontological literature, but we suggest that a new direction has already taken place in our contemporary era, and this new direction (a change on the curve—the [5.0] inflection point) does not simply overturn or replace the *scientific management of ageing*, but rather has changed via a metamorphosis in perspective and outcome into a "scientific-technological" *Weltanschauung* seeking to move beyond ageing as a necessary stage in the life course; rather ageing (biologically, socially, and psychologically) is something to be overcome and transcended, incrementally, and thus completely.

We further propose that another related, but vastly different trajectory of epistemological, ontological, and experiential approaches to ageing will soon eclipse the supposed penultimate goal (in our limited temporal horizon) of *optimal ageing* in gerontology. In other words, the momentum has shifted and the scientific activity within ageing is undergoing a transformation. The driving force in gerontology will no longer be a descriptive analysis of the "longevity revolution" (Butler 2008; Greenbaum 2010), but a proscriptive call to action in the implementation and practice of making extreme *longevity* no longer revolutionary, but normative and customary. And along with "normative" longevity will then come the expected [5.0] change—toward a "post ageing".

Therefore, we are proposing a significant change in the present curvature and that there is another significant shift in the literature ahead. Will optimal ageing [4.0] and ageing as challenge [3.0] and ageing as problem [2.0] and ageing with reflection [1.0] still continue to influence the literature? Yes… *of course*. But we propose that these previous tracks of prevailing themes have already reached their zenith in terms of the cumulative effect of research momentum and activity, curriculum content and delivery, and public interest. Of course, there will always be enough rooms in the large house that is gerontology for the philosophy of ageing [1.0] and the understanding of the social construction of ageing—and for a humanistic gerontology. But the soon-to-be *largest* room in the house, where the greatest proportion of interest and activity and exponential growth will take place, is the area where *bioengineering* and *technology* are discussed, showcased, and subsequently transform the significance of the ageing experience.

This proposed inflection point—this new tip of the spear in research, teaching, and application—is already underway; and, although such a claim may appear to be grandiloquent to those fully invested in their own research specialties and thematic tracks and service sectors that represent previous inflection points, we submit that the new transformation will be tectonic in scope and that the ripple effect will influence the very nature of our understanding of the ageing experience.

Butler's (2008) book, *The Longevity Revolution* (see also review of book by Finch 2009), and the edited book by Greenbaum (2010) *Longevity Rules: How to Age Well Into the Future*, in our estimation, represent the culmination of the positive derivative (for inflection [4.0]) that has described and analyzed the deepening human condition influenced by the radical transitions associated with the exceptional and "unprecedented demographic transformation" (Butler 2008, p. xi) in the 20th century. We propose that it is also a part of a hermeneutical inflection point representative of a new direction in the ageing experience that will be increasingly directed by the monumental advancements in bioengineering and in bio-technology. This inflection point is summarized in the statement from the International Longevity Center (ILC) (2008) taken from their annual report "Embracing Longevity",

> We recognize longevity as a great human and social achievement that can only advance if we embrace it fully in all of its dimensions through knowledge, action and creative solutions.

And so while the scientific management of ageing and the drive towards an optimal ageing continues to generate energy for the wheels of normative science, we are suggesting that we are already moving into a *post ageing* era [5.0] inspired and being directed by the realm of *bio-techno-engineering*, which will overtake and proceed beyond the domain of optimal ageing [4.0]. Indeed, the [4.0] inflection point with its goal of ageing as a *reward* has served as precursor, a sentinel, and a harbinger. This post ageing *Weltanschauung* has the capacity to transform all aspects of existential and humanistic meaning of the ageing experience in the future (see also Kirby 2009). If anything, we are convinced that Cole's concerns about the dominion of "scientific management of ageing" will pale in comparison to what is to come in the 21st century.

2.6 [4.0] Reviewing the Current and Triumphal Positive Derivative in the Field of Ageing

Before we present the evidence and the case for the next inflection point [5.0] of "post ageing", ageing as an artifact, let us briefly review the current proposed positive derivative (and the curvature) that represents optimal ageing [4.0]. In our current line of theoretical and conceptual understanding of ageing, we have witnessed not only an increased longevity but also an increased expectation that all will live not only longer but also significantly and substantially *better*.

We have quickly moved from contemplating a demographic revolution of "squaring the pyramid" (Pifer and Bronte 1986a) to the promotion of a "longevity revolution" (Butler 2008; Roszak 2001) in just a few decades. It appears that the Stoic tradition of embracing the shortness of life is but a quaint view from yesteryear, and that the concerns of population ageing (Siegel and Taeuber 1986) have been transformed into a philosophical attitude that we can "have our cake and eat it too".

It used to be said that *life is short and art is long*; but in our high point for the era of the "scientific management of ageing" (Cole 1992) our goal is now the art of living longer, and *optimally so.* As Silvertown (2014) points out, "over the last two centuries our own species has increased its average life span by nearly a quarter". Our current landscape for understanding the experience of ageing is represented by the following indicators of the "received view" which illustrate but do not exhaust the examples in the literature: *age wave* (Dychtwald 1990); *fountain of age* (Friedan 1993); *from age-ing to sage-ing* (Schachter-Shalomi 1997) and that we have entered into phase of *age power* (Dychtwald 1999), and the power years, (Dychtwald and Kadlec 2005); *the creative age* (Cohen 2001); *third age* (Sadler 2000); *successful ageing* (Rowe and Kahn 1999); *prime time* (Freedman 2000); and *encore* (Freedman 2007); *ageing well* (Valliant 2002); *positive ageing* (Hill 2005); *healthy ageing* (Weil 2007); *the art of ageing* (Nuland 2007); *productive ageing* (Morrow-Howell et al. 2001); *transcendence in later life* (Tornstam 1999–2000); *vital ageing* (Achenbaum 2005); *self-empowerment* (Maples and Abney 2006); *elder culture* (Roszak 2009); and *ageing well* (Greenbaum 2010).

These indicators represent a collective premise (not a paradigm) that captures the essence of optimal ageing [4.0] as the prevailing theme in gerontology. It is the resulting effect of previous inflection points that have guided the scholarship of ageing. Thus we are in agreement with Bass and Ferraro (2000) that gerontology is yet again in transition, but we do not forecast an evolving paradigm or the possibility of an emergent discipline for gerontology. Our field will sustain itself in a more robust way as "interdisciplinary" by letting go of the need to identify a paradigm, per se, for the field. The evolution that is taking place in our field is a highly complex set of interrelated threads of scholarship representing previous prevailing themes that increase (along a curvature with time passing) as a positive derivative, but with a change in direction along the curve. The change is due to intersecting forces within and outside of the permeable boundary for gerontology, which is the quite natural effect of the interdisciplinary foundation and operation that is gerontology. Our science and our inquiries into the ageing experience are influenced by the operations and activities from other fields, specialties, disciplines, and organizations. They too are investigating the domain of "ageing"—and many of their activities represent "sentinel" operations that "mainstream" gerontology or those engaged in normative science (or "puzzle-solving" as Kuhn called it) are simply not aware of or ignore because it does not fit their assumptions. Although Kuhn described the process of "revolutionary science" as the break point set against "normal science", it appears to me that in gerontology, there is more of an ascent and then gradual flattening of one predominant theme, while other themes emerge and enter the landscape of potential inflection points. A select idea will gather momentum and critical mass, and rise as a different (but positive) increase against the previous curvature. There does not appear to be any revolutionary "flip" or "break point" in gerontology. Our field is simply too broad and too interconnected with other disciplinary ventures and professions to have one pristine "gerontological paradigm" dominate the field. Although there is the distinct possibility, in fact the probability, that there may be a bona fide paradigm to refer to in other connected fields or disciplines, gerontology will be driven less by shifts dependent on revolutionary science than it will be by shifts due to inflection points. These inflection points do not replace the existing order but rather build upon it, and then change in direction from the previous arc in curvature (see also Agamben 2009). We have a *prevailing theme* (a meta-theoretical position) serving as an implied "lodestar", a *raison d'être*. In the current manifestation of the curvature, we have reached the zenith of optimal ageing [4.0] which—and let us be clear here—will continue to be a research track, a publication category, a curriculum offering, a service mission, and "quasi-paradigm" for some in the field. In effect, this also means that we have taken the "meaning" of later life to be more—that is, we want to be productive, vital, successful, positive, and as engaged as before (that is before ageing "took place"). There is no stoic acceptance or resignation or revolt, only the conquering of all that represents senescence. We have elected to have it reframed, re-packaged and re-tooled to become an anti-senescence. We don't retire, we re-career. We don't age, we transcend. We don't decline, we transform. We pay homage to Longevity as the Prince, but the ultimate loyalty is to Immortality as the King.

So, perhaps we have not quite reached the destination of human progression in relation to the ageing experience. Is there something more to be gained and achieved *beyond* optimal ageing, which could completely transcend the ageing experience altogether? The next inflection point [5.0] is labeled *Post Ageing*, reflecting an array of technologies and bioengineering that could forever alter the landscape of life's journey. We propose that humanity is crossing the threshold into the next positive derivative.

2.7 [5.0] Post Ageing, or Ageing as an Artifact

The metaphysical traditions and reflections of Seneca and Marcus Aurelius have been turned on their head so that we now assume life can never be *long enough.* The only time we are wasting in our modern/postmodern condition is by not allowing or supporting the scientific and technological movement in being *fast enough* in the quest for a "post ageing" condition and the possibility of removing the "final constraint" of existence, death itself. We may think of death as inevitable, but it has also become more of a nuisance than a fulcrum for existential significance and metaphysical reflection.

What is wanted now is the active investigation and implementation of strategies and tactics that will create a longer and longer interval between birth and death (see Greenbaum 2010)—with the ultimate goal of *post ageing*. Scientists and researchers differ on what they believe has brought us this far, to this level of longevity. However, we believe we will come to see this inflection point and resulting curvature as the prevailing theme within gerontology, and with it the socio-cultural expectation that science and technology continue to serve as the catalyst for optimal ageing transforming into post ageing. Many will see this a necessary transition, as an entitlement for simply being alive—so that having a life can be extended for as long as possible with minimal ageing, or ultimately with no manifestations of ageing at all.

But before you think this is all irrational exuberance on our part (and others who share our perspective), we want the reader to realize that we are aware of the many daunting issues that would counter any post ageing [5.0] scenario. We too can appreciate and understand the contra-scenarios suggested by others (see Peterson 1999) who see living in a world of increasing Methuselahs who are *beyond ageing* and would thus contribute to some hellish context, which would result in diminishing the quality of life for almost everyone else—*both economically and environmentally*. We do acknowledge that any notion of a "post ageing" could be seen as representing ageism, or as a titanic denial (see Gillick 2006), or discounting any possibilities of "shortgevity" (Butler 2008), or ignoring the realities of an "ageing world" that sees demographic ageing and its attendant "problems and challenges" (representative of [2.0] and [3.0] themes) as a "slow burning fuse" (see special report from *The Economist*, June 27, 2009). However, while there is cause for considerable concern about many issues, as Schulz and Binstock (2006) have shown, with smart individual choices and a variety of sound policies and programs in place, the elderly could prosper and a demographic tsunami does not become inevitable (see also Hudson 2009). Nevertheless, we will cite just a few examples that illustrate substantial threats to sustaining *optimal ageing* as our current prevailing theme in gerontology and serve as possible barriers to the realization of *post ageing* as the prevailing theme in our future.

2.8 Perceived Barriers to Change

As previously mentioned, the "ageing as challenge" [3.0] theme has generated important research findings that investigate the demographic transitions from various levels—from the city block and census track level to the other end of the scale at the global level (see Christensen et al. 2009; Crampton 2009; Uhlenberg 2009). This has led to some innovative re-conceptualizations of both the meaning (and definition) of *age* and *ageing* to better understand and compare people who live in periods and places where life expectancies differ by using the concept of "prospective age" (Sanderson and Scherbov 2008). For example, Fonseca and colleagues (2012), in their dynamic stochastic model of health production, assume in their baseline that "agents suffering from chronic conditions have access to better care, and optimally choose to spend more on medical care". This model, as expected, subsequently predicts that "life expectancy should continue to rise despite the noted increase in the prevalence of chronic conditions". Yet the disparities in health, as evidenced from the data generated from various parts of the world, are of great concern. They indicate that not only is increased longevity not a given universal expectation but also that "shortgevity" may indeed be the reality for many geographic areas across the globe, including some areas within the United States, due to a myriad of conditions that affect health status and the quality of life.

For example, in a recent study by the Robert Wood Johnson Foundation (2009), "Reaching America's Health Potential Among Adults: A State-by-State Look at Adult Health," it was found that almost half of all adults 25–74 in the United States reported being in less than very good health, and that the rate differed depending on one's level of education. Adults who did not graduate from high school are more than two and half times as likely to be in less than very good health as college graduates. Those who graduated from high school but not college are nearly twice as likely to be in less than very good health as college graduates. This specific study revealed

> substantial shortfalls in the health of American adults at the national level as well as in every state. Shortfalls in health are greatest among the most-disadvantaged adults, but even those considered middle class are less healthy than adults with greater social and economic advantages (p. 3).

These findings obviously highlight a major concern that *optimal ageing*—and for that matter any potential *post ageing* experience—may be limited to a *select group of people* who have "greater social and economic advantages". Geographic patterns of disparities in mental health across the U.S. indicate significant variations in unmet mental health care needs (Moriarty et al. 2009). They also reveal spatial patterns of natural hazards mortality in the United States (Borden and Cutter 2008). Both of these patterns point to a greater need for preventive measures in emergency planning, a strengthening in the public health sector, and an educational awareness for all socio-economic groups—particularly those most vulnerable, including older adults without social capital. We have learned that a concentrated effort in this country to reduce fine-particulate air pollution has resulted in increased life expectancy (Pope et al. 2009), which is an "across-the-board" dividend for all age groups from the enforcement of environmental protections; yet as Ezzati et al. (2008) have reported in their study on trends in county mortality and cross-county mortality disparities, including the contributions of specific diseases to county level mortality trends, there was a steady *increase in mortality inequality* across US counties between 1983 and 1999 as a result of stagnation and even increase in mortality among the worst-off segment of the population. Female mortality increased in a large number of counties, primarily because of chronic diseases related to smoking, overweight/obesity, and high blood pressure. So while *optimal ageing* [4.0] may be the current prevailing theme and predominant goal in gerontology, there are still serious social, cultural, public health, and environmental conditions that create and sustain disparities across the human life course (see also Frey et al. 2009). The investigation, intervention, and hoped for prevention of these disparities not only represents a continuation of the [3.0] and [2.0] curvatures of research, teaching, and practice as it relates to the ageing experience (see Institute of Medicine 2009, report, "Retooling for an Ageing America: Building the Health Care Workforce"), but is imperative so that these issues of inequalities by race, ethnicity, class, and geographic region are adequately addressed *before* we claim that optimal ageing is the normative experience for older adults (see Glymour et al. 2009). It is one thing to state that optimal ageing is the prevailing theme and predominant goal, but it is another to then state that it is the prevailing and expected *experience* for the majority of older adults in this country. Thus, while the optimization of ageing is the prevailing theme in gerontology and serves as the current lodestar for the longevity revolution that is underway, there is also the need to see it as the *expected* experience toward the latter part of the journey of life, for all citizens.

Another concern is the expectation from the public that to experience a triple-digit chronological age experience is practically an entitlement. With this regard, we need to heed the wisdom of Hall (2008) in an editorial in the *Archives of Internal Medicine*, who offered that,

> Of course longevity is a Pyrrhic victory if those additional years are characterized by inexorable morbidity from chronic illness, frailty-associated disability, and increasingly lowered quality of life (p. 262).

In other words, the continued momentum for the optimization of ageing [4.0] and the subsequent emergence of the [5.0] post ageing curvature is very much dependent on the continuation of biological and medical research (see Michel et al. 2008; Norris et al. 2007). This research into the issues of senescence and the policy issues regarding health care for older Americans with multiple chronic conditions, is vital in continuing to compress morbidity and disability "into a smaller time frame near the end of life as predicted by Fries in the 'compression of morbidity' hypothesis" (Hall 2008, p. 263).

Yet, despite these potential gaps in the sustained momentum of *optimal ageing* [4.0] and the emergence of a *post ageing* [5.0] curvature, there is also evidence that the overall experience of "growing old in America" is summarized in this statement: *the older people get, the younger they feel* (Pew Research Center 2009). Interestingly, this landmark study found significant generational differences in the expectations and realities of the ageing experience. The share of younger and middle-aged adults who report expecting to encounter potential problems related to old age is much *higher* than the share of older adults who report actually experiencing them. Our point here is that the actual experiences of older adults is better than what most people realize, and that not only is there a compression of morbidity, there also appears to be a compression of the "feeling" of senescence into the later years of life. This sense runs parallel to the notion that, in general, *ageing can be optimized* up to a point, which appears to be (according to this survey) approximately the age of 90. After that point, the expectations for any significant *quality of life* (optimal ageing) are significantly lowered.

But this issue of "living to a good old age"—whether that be 85, 90, or 115 years—represents a cogent segue into the next dimension of this book. That is, is there a realistic possibility that not only can age be optimized into the ninth decade (see Greenbaum 2010), but also for life to be extended, *and optimized*, beyond that? Can we, given the expansion and growth of bioengineering and technology, contemplate an aggressive life extension beyond the centenarian mark into the decades that follow? Can we expect that there will be dramatic successes in optimizing ageing with anti-ageing medicine? Or with nanotechnology? Or with biotechnology?

Is it even possible that we should contemplate—and thus pursue—the possibility of immortality in our lifetimes? Will we move beyond ageing itself into the realm of a *post ageing* curvature [5.0]?

2.9 Ending Ageing

We are suggesting that this change in direction, this new positive derivative (see Adler 2012) for the *investigation, understanding,* and *experiencing* of ageing will be driven, guided, and fueled by the intersect of the theory and research associated with biotechnology, computer technology, and molecular biology (Critser 2010; Liu et al. 2014; Stipp 2010; Weiner 2010). One could argue that these intersecting influences on the study of ageing may simply represent an extension of *optimal ageing* (thus, a [4.1] version), but we will argue that the goal in this new theme is simply *not* to optimize ageing, but rather to surpass it, to transcend it, *to end it*. The theme that will emerge is to move beyond ageing so that the cultural history, the existential landscape, and the humanistic interpretation thereof will all be dramatically transformed by what Nicholas Carr (2008) referred to as the "the big switch," what Kirby referred to as "digimodernism," what Pettman (2006) referred to as "techtonics", and Joel Garreau (2005) referred to as a "radical evolution" in the human condition. Garreau (2005) proposes that these new technologies will offer both promise and peril in the enhancement of our minds, bodies, "and what it means to be human" (see also Mehlman 2009). We further propose that the *future of gerontology* will be in embracing this new inflection point [5.0]—and that the study of ageing will undergo a change in direction in guiding research, teaching, and practice. As we have stated before in this book, previous themes from other inflection points continue onward in gerontology as focal points for some scholars in the field, but each subsequent inflection point is understood in terms of becoming the primary guide for the field: its *raison d'être*. Thus, optimal ageing will continue as a theme, but we propose that it will yield to the next inflection point (and resulting curvature) that is now underway. We will end this section with a few excerpts to set the stage for what we propose is the next inflection point in gerontology and the study of ageing—[5.0]: Post Ageing (ageing as an *artifact*). We propose that the initial signs and the sentinel activities are already in place, giving us a preliminary look into the new direction:

> There will soon be as many artificial neurons on earth, in all of our 'intelligent' machines, as in all our 'natural' brains (120 billion neurons each). Are we not running the risk, after the elimination of dark matter, of an exhaustion of all grey matter, from the point when the stock of Artificial Intelligence exceeds the symbolic capital of the species, this latter ceasing to exist once it's much more efficient artificial counterpart comes into being? Is there room on the earth for as many artificial as natural species, for as much computer-generated substance as organic matter, dead or alive, for as much Artificial Intelligence as natural intelligence? Is there room for the world and its double?
> —Jean Baudrillard (2005). *The Intelligence of Evil or the Lucidity Pact*. Berg: New York. p. 193–194.

> Two revolutions will affect the well-being of older Americans in the twenty-first century: the demographic revolution of an ageing society and the scientific revolution of molecular biology.
> —Catherine Read, Robert C. Green, Michael Smyer (Eds.) (2008). *Ageing, Technology, and the Future,* The Johns Hopkins University Press. Baltimore, MD. p. xi.

> It is possible that we are now entering a new Romantic Age, extending over the first half of the twenty-first century, with the technological billionaires of today playing roles similar to the enlightened aristocrats of the 18th century?… If this new Romantic Age is real, it will be centered on biology and computers, as the old one was centered on chemistry and poetry.
> —Freeman Dyson (2009). When Science and Poetry Were Friends. New York Review of Books. August 13, 2009 (#13) [a review of the book: *The Age of Wonder: How the Romantic Generation Discovered the Beauty and Terror of Science* by Richard Holmes. Pantheon]

> To the reader of 2009, some of these changes {biotechnology} may sound freaky or unsettling. But a century from now, they'll seem as normal as pacemakers, hip replacements and in vitro fertilization have become today. Our descendants, like us, won't just be technology's judges. They'll be its products too.
> —William Saletan (2009). *You: The updated owner's manual*. New York Times Book Review. Crossroads—A Series of Essays. August 2, 2009; p. 23.

References

Achenbaum, A. (2001). Productive ageing in historical context. In N. Morrow-Howell, J. Hinterlong & M. Sherraden (Eds.), *Productive ageing; concepts and challenges* (pp. 19–35). Baltimore, MD: Johns Hopkins University Press.

Achenbaum, A. (2005). *Older Americans, vital communities: A bold vision for societal ageing*. Baltimore, MD: The Johns Hopkins University Press.

Adler, F. R. (2012). *Modeling the dynamics of life: Calculus and probability for life scientists* (3rd ed.). Independence, KY: Cengage Learning.

Agamben, G. (2009). *The signature of all things*. New York: Zone Books.

Alexander, H. (2009). Reflections on Benjamin Button. *Philosophy and Literature, 33*, 1–17.

Alkema, G., & Alley, D. (2006). Gerontology's future: An integrative model for disciplinary advancement. *The Gerontologist, 46*, 574–582.

Amery, J. (1994). *On ageing: Revolt and resignation*. Bloomington, IL: University of Illinois Press.

Barzun, J. (2000). *From dawn to decadence: 1500 to the present*. New York: Harper Collins Publishers.

Bass, S. A. (2007). The power of persistence in shaping gerontological thought and practice. *Journal of Ageing and Social Policy, 19*(3), 133–142.

Bass, S. A., & Ferraro, K. (2000). Gerontology education in transition: Considering disciplinary and paradigmatic evolution. *The Gerontologist, 40*(1), 97–106.

Berlin, I. (1990). *The crooked timber of humanity*. Princeton, NJ: Princeton University Press.

Bongaarts, J. (2009). Trends in senescent life expectancy. *Population Studies, 63*(3), 203–213.

Borden, K. A. & Cutter, S. (2008). Spatial patterns of natural hazards mortality in the United States. *International Journal of Health Geographics, 7*(64). Available at http://www.ij-healthgeographics.com

Buettner, D. (2008). *The blue zones: Lessons for living longer from the people who've lived the longest*. Washington, DC: National Geographic Magazine.

Butler, R. (1975). *Why survive? Being old in America*. New York: Harper & Row.

Butler, R. (2008). *The longevity revolution: The benefits and challenges of living a long life*. New York: Public Affairs.

Butler, R. N., & Lewis, M. I. (1973). *Ageing and mental health: Positive psychosocial approaches*. St. Louis, MO: The C.V. Mosby Company.

Carr, N. (2008). Is google making us stupid? What the internet is doing to our brains. *The Atlantic*, (July/August). Available at http://www.theatlantic.com/doc/200807/google

Charney, M. (2009). *Wrinkled deep in time: Ageing in Shakespeare*. New York: Columbia University Press.

Christensen, K., Doblhammer, G., Rau, R., & Vaupel, J. (2009). Ageing populations: The challenges ahead. *The Lancet, 374*, 1196–1208.

Cohen, G. (2001). *The creative age: Awakening human potential in the second half of life*. New York: Harper Paperbacks.

Cole, T. R. (1992). *The journey of life: A cultural history of ageing in America*. New York: Cambridge University Press.

Cole, T. R., Kastenbaum, R., & Ray, R. (Eds.). (2000). *Handbook of the humanities and ageing*. New York: Springer.

Cole, T. R., Ray, R., & Kastenbaum, R. (2010). *A guide to humanistic studies in ageing: What does it mean to grow old?*. Baltimore, MD: The Johns Hopkins University Press.

Cole, T. R., & Sierpina, M. (2007). Humanistic gerontology and the meanings of ageing. In J. M. Wilmoth & K. F. Ferraro (Eds.), *Gerontology: Perspectives and issues* (3rd ed., pp. 245–264). New York: Springer.

Cole, T. R., & Winkler, M. G. (Eds.). (1994). *The Oxford book of ageing: Reflections on the journey of life*. New York: Oxford University Press.

Comfort, A. (1964). *The ageing of senescence*. New York: Holt, Rinehart and Winston, Inc. (first published in 1956 as *The Biology of Senescence*).

Comfort, A. (1976). *A good age*. New York: Crown Publishers.

Crampton, A. (2009). *Global ageing: Emerging challenges*. The Pardee Papers. No. 6. Boston: Boston University. Available at http://www.bu/edu/pardee

Critser, G. (2010). *Eternity soup: Inside the quest to end ageing*. New York: Harmony Books.

de Beauvior, S. (1972). *The coming of age*. New York: G.P. Putnam.

Dychtwald, K. (1990). *The age wave: How the most important trend of our time can change your future*. New York: Bantam.

Dychtwald, K. (1999). *Age power: How the 21st century will be ruled by the new old*. New York: Tarcher.

Dychtwald, K., & Kadlec, D. (2005). *The power years: A user's guide to the rest of your life*. New York: John Wiley and Sons.
Dyson, F. (2009). *When science and poetry were friends*. New York: Review of Books.
Edman, I. (Ed.). (1928). *The philosophy of schopenhauer*. New York: The Modern Library.
Eisdorfer, C., & Powell Lawton, M. P. (1973). *The psychology of adult development and ageing*. Washington, DC: American Psychological Association.
Estes, C. (1979). *The ageing enterprise*. San Francisco: Jossey-Bass.
Estes, C. (1993). The ageing enterprise revisited. *The Gerontologist, 33*(3), 292–297.
Ezzati, M., Friedman, A. B., Kulkarni, S. C., & Murray, C. J. (2008). The reversal of fortunes: Trends in county mortality and cross-county mortality disparities in the United States. *PLoS Med, 5*(4), e66. doi:10.1371/journal.pmed.0050066.
Ferraro, K. (2006). Imagining the disciplinary advancement of gerontology: Whither the tipping point? *The Gerontologist, 46*(5), 571–573.
Finch, C. (2009). The gerevolutions of Bob Butler. *The Gerontologist, 49*(4), 577–579.
Flanagan, O. (2002). *The problem of the soul*. New York: Basic Books.
Fonseca, R., Gaudette, E., Michaud, P. (2012) *Forecasting population health, health spending, and mortality*. Mimeo presented in 46th Canadian Economics Association (CEA) Conference. 6 August 2012, Calgary, Canada.
Freedman, M. (2000). *Prime time: How baby boomers will revolutionize retirement and transform America*. Cambridge: Perseus Books Group.
Freedman, M. (2007). *Encore: Finding work that matters in the second half of life*. Cambridge: Perseus Books Group.
Frey, W., Berube, A., Singer, A., & Wilson, J. (2009). *Getting current: Recent demographic trends in metropolitan america*. The Brookings Institute. Available at http://www.brookings.edu/reports/2009/03_metro_demographic_trends.aspx
Friedan, B. (1993). *The fountain of age*. New York: Simon & Schuster.
Garreau, J. (2005). *Radical evolution: The promise and peril of enhancing our minds, our bodies—and what it means to be human*. New York: Broadway (Random House).
Gilbert, M. (2001). *History of the twentieth century*. New York: Harper Collins Publishers.
Gillick, M. R. (2006). *The denial of ageing: Perpetual youth, eternal life, and other dangerous fantasies*. Cambridge, MA: Harvard University Press.
Glymour, N. M., Kosheleva, A., & Boden-Albala, B. (2009). Birth and adult residence in the Stoke Belt independently predict stroke mortality. *Neurology, 73*, 1858–1865.
Goldsmith, J. (2008). *The long baby boom: An optimistic vision for a graying generation*. Baltimore, MD: The Johns Hopkins University Press.
Gottlieb, A. (2002). *The dream of reason: A history of philosophy from the greeks to the renaissance*. New York: W.W. Norton & Co.
Greenbaum, S. (2010). *Longevity rules: How to age well into the future*. Sacramento, CA: Eskaton.
Haber, D. (2009). Gerontology: Adding an empowerment paradigm. *Journal of Applied Gerontology, 28*(3), 283–297.
Hall, S. G. (1922). *Senescence: The last half of life*. New York: D. Appleton & Co.
Hall, W. J. (2008). Centenarians: Metaphor becomes reality. *Archives of Internal Medicine, 168*(3), 262–263.
Halter, J. B., Ouslander, J. G., Tinetti, M. E., Studenski, S., High, K. P., Asthana, S., et al. (2009). *Hazzard's geriatric medicine and gerontology: Principles of geriatric medicine and gerontology* (6th ed.). New York: McGraw-Hill Professional.
Hannan, B. (2009). *The riddle of the world: A reconsideration of schopenhauer's philosophy*. New York: Oxford University Press.
Hayflick, L. (1994). *How and why we age*. New York: Ballantine Books.
Hill, R. (2005). *Positive ageing: A guide for mental health professionals and consumers*. New York: W. W. Norton & Co.
Holmes, R. (2009). *The age of wonder: How the romantic generation discovered the beauty and terror of science*. New York: Harper Collins.

Hudson, R. B. (2009). *Boomer bust? Economic and political issues of the graying society.* (Volume 1: Perspectives on the boomers; Volume 2: The boomers and their future.) Westport, CT: Praeger Publishing.

Institute of Medicine (2009). *Retooling for an ageing America: Building the health care workforce.* Institute of Medicine of the National Academies. Washington, DC: National Academy Press.

International Longevity Center (ILC-USA). (2008). *Embracing Longevity: Annual Report 2008.* New York. Available at http://www.ilcusa.org

International Longevity Center Global Alliance. (2009). *Global ageing report: Threats to longevity, A call to action.* New York. Available at http://www.ilc-alliance.org

Jung, C. (1933). *Modern man in search of soul.* New York: Harcourt, Brace and Company.

Kinsella, K., & He, W. (2009). *An ageing world: 2008 (P95/09-1).* Washington, DC: U.S. Census Bureau and National Institute of Ageing.

Kirby, A. (2009). *Digimodernism: How new technologies dismantle the postmodern and reconfigure our culture.* New York: Continuum.

Krause, N. (2009). Meaning in life and mortality. *The Journals of Gerontology Series B: Psychological Sciences and Social Sciences, 64B*(4), 517–527.

Kronos Longevity Research Institute (KLRI). (2009). *Gray is the new gold—Optimism in ageing research.* Available at http://www.knronosinstitute.org

Liu, Y., He, Y., Zhang, Y., Cai, W., Yang, L., & Xu, L. et al. (2014). Absence of A673T variant in APP gene indicates an alternative protective mechanism contributing to longevity in Chinese individuals. *Neurobiology of Ageing, 35*, 935e11–935e12.

Magee, B. (1997). *The philosophy of Schopenhauer.* New York: Oxford University Press.

Maples, M. F., & Abney, P. C. (2006). Baby boomers mature and gerontological counseling comes of age. *Journal of Counseling and Development, 84*, 3–9.

Matthewman, S., & Hoey, D. (2006). What happened to postmodernism? *Sociology, 40*(3), 529–547.

Mehlman, M. J. (2009). *The price of perfection: Individualism and society in the era of biomedical enhancement.* Baltimore, MD: The Johns Hopkins University Press.

Michel, J., Newton, J., & Kirkwood, T. (2008). Medical challenges of improving the quality of a longer life. *JAMA, 299*(6), 688–690.

Moody, H. (2004/2005). Silver Industries and the new ageing enterprise. *Generations*, Winter. Available at http://www.generationsjounral.org/generations/gen28-4/article.cfm

Moody, H. (2008). *The new ageing enterprise. Occasional papers, # 4.* Washington DC: AARP Academic Affairs.

Moriarty, D., Zack, M., Holt, J. B., Chapman, D., & Safran, M. (2009). Geographic patterns of frequent mental distress. *American Journal of Preventative Medicine, 36*(6), 497–505.

Morrow-Howell, N., Hinterlong, J., & Sherraden, M. (Eds.). (2001). *Productive ageing: Concerns and challenges.* Baltimore, MD: The Johns Hopkins University Press.

Norris, S., High, K., Gill, T., Hennessy, S., Kutner, J., Reuben, D., et al. (2007). Health care for older Americans with multiple chronic conditions: A research agenda. *Journal of Americans Geriatrics Society, 56*, 149–159.

Nuland S. B. (2007). *The art of ageing: A doctor's prescription for well-being.* New York: Random House.

Olshansky, S. J., & Carnes, B. (2001). *The quest for immortality: Science at the frontiers of ageing.* New York: W. W. Norton & Co.

Olshansky, S. J., & Carnes, B. A. (2009). The future of longevity. In P. Uhlenberg (Ed.), *International handbook of population ageing* (pp. 731–745). New York: Springer.

Olshansky, S. J., Goldman, D. P., Zheng, Y., & Rowe, J. (2009). Ageing in America in the twenty-first century: demographic forecasts from the MacArthur Foundation research network on an ageing society. *The Milbank Quarterly, 87*(4), 842–862.

Peterson, P. (1999). Gray dawn: The global ageing crisis. *Foreign Affairs*, Jan/Feb. Available at http://www.foreignaffairs.com/articles/54620/peter-g-peterson/gray-dawn-the-global-ageing-crisis

Pettman, D. (2006). *Love and other technologies: Retrofitting eros for the information age*. New York: Fordham University Press.

Pew Research Center. (2009). *Growing old in America: Expectations vs. reality*. Pew Research Center. Available at http://pewsocialtrends.org

Pifer, A. & Bronte, L. (1986a). Introduction: Squaring the pyramid. *Daedalus, Winter, The Ageing Society, 115*(1), 1–11. Proceedings of the American Academy Arts and Sciences, New York.

Pifer, A., & Bronte, L. (1986b). *Our ageing society: Paradox and promise*. New York: W. W. Norton & Company.

Pope, C. A., Ezzati, M., & Dockery, D. W. (2009). Fine-particulate air pollution and life expectancy in the United States. *The New England Journal of Medicine, 360*(4), 376–386.

Porter, R. (2003). *Flesh in the age of reason: The modern foundations of body and soul*. New York: W.W. Norton & Co.

Posner, R. A. (1995). Ageing *and old age*.Chicago, IL: University of Chicago Press.

Preston, S., & Ho, J. Y. (2009). *Low life expectancy in the United States: Is the health care system at fault?* PSC Working Paper Series PSC 09-03. Available at http://repository.upenn.edu/psc_working_papers/13

Pruchno, R. A., & Smyer, M. A. (Eds.). (2007). *Challenges of an ageing society: Ethical dilemmas, political issues*. Baltimore, MD: The Johns Hopkins University Press.

Quinodoz, D. (2010). *Growing old: A journey of self-discovery*. New York: Routledge.

Robert Wood Johnson Foundation. (2009). Reaching America's health potential among adults: A state-by-state look at adult health. Available at http://www.rwjf.org

Robine, J. M., Jagger, C., & Crimmins, E. (Eds.). (2013). *Healthy longevity, a global approach. Annual review of gerontology and geriatrics, 33*. New York: Springer.

Roszak, T. (1998). *America the wise: The longevity revolution and the true wealth of nations*. Boston: Houton Mifflin, Co.

Roszak, T. (2001). *Longevity revolution: As boomers become elders*. Chicago: Berkeley Hills Books.

Roszak, T. (2009). *The making of an elder culture: Reflections on the future of America's most audacious generation*. Gabriola Island, BC, Canada: New Society Publishers.

Rowe, J. W., & Kahn, R. L. (1999). *Successful ageing*. New York: Dell Publishing.

Sadler, W. A. (2000). *The third age: 6 principles for growth and renewal after forty*. Boston: Da Capo Press.

Sanderson, W., & Scherbov, S. (2008). Rethinking age and ageing. *Population Bulletin, 63*(4), 3–16.

Schachter-Shalomi, Z. (1997). *From age-ing to sage-ing: A profound new vision of growing older*. New York: Warner Books.

Schopenhauer, A. (2008). (T.B. Saunders, Trans.). *The wisdom of life and counsels and maxims*. Digireads.com Publishing. ISBN 1420931121, 9781420931129.

Schulz, J. H., & Binstock, R. H. (2006). *Ageing nation: The economics and politics of growing older in America*. Westport, CT: Praeger.

Sheehy, G. (1996). *New passages: Mapping your life across time*. New York: Random House.

Siegel, J. & Taeuber, C. (1986). Demographic perspectives on the long-lived society. *Daedalus, Winter, The Ageing Society, 115*(1), 77–117. Proceedings of the American Academy Arts and Sciences, New York.

Silvertown, J. (2014). *The long and the short of it*. Chicago IL: University of Chicago Press.

Stipp, D. (2010). *The youth pill: Scientists at the brink of an anti-ageing revolution*. New York: Current (Penguin).

Taylor, C. (2007). *A secular age*. Cambridge, MA: The Belknap Press of Harvard University Press.

Tornstam, L. (2000). Transcendence in later life. *Generations, 23*(4), 10–14.

Torres-Gil, F. (1992). *The new ageing: Politics and change in America*. Boston: Auburn House.

Uhlenberg, P. (Ed.). (2009). *International handbook of population ageing*. New York: Springer.

Valliant, G. (2002). *Ageing well: Surprising guideposts to a happier life from the landmark Harvard study of adult development*. Boston: Little Brown.

Warthin, A. S. (1930). *Old age: The Major involution—The physiology and pathology of the ageing process*. New York: Paul B. Hoeber Inc.

Weil, A. (2007). *Healthy ageing: A lifelong guide to your well-being*. New York: Random House.

Weiner, J. (2010). *Long for this world: The strange science of immortality*. New York: Harper Collins.

Weiss, R. S., & Bass, S. (Eds.). (2002). *Challenges of the third age: Meaning and purpose in later life*. New York: Oxford University Press.

Wright, S. D. (2008). Life in the long lane—a review essay on the longevity revolution: The benefits and challenges of living a long life by Robert N. Butler. *Journal of the American Heart Association*, *2*(3/4), 298–313.

Part II
Toward Post Ageing: A Critical Examination and Provisional Typology for Understanding the Varied Roles of Technology in an Ageing Society

Chapter 3
[5.0] Post Ageing

Abstract To reinterpret the developments and shifts in gerontology from an historical perspective (in hindsight) by using inflection points is one thing, but to offer a prospective prevailing theme (such as [5.0]) before any critical mass has taken place to verify and corroborate the theme actually exists is bound to be a risky venture, a conjecture, even an adventure. But such is the purpose of this book: to tread carefully, but with courage and integrity, so as to look ahead and create the profile for what we think is the next inflection point in gerontological research, teaching, and application.

Keywords Assistive technology · Bioengineering · Gerotechnology · GRIN technologies · Post-modernism · Themes in gerontology

We have proposed that we consider *inflection points* as the more appropriate structure to understand changes in prevailing themes in gerontology as opposed to the Kuhnian notion of "paradigm" or "paradigm shifts." We do not take exception to the Kuhnian stance to a philosophy of science, we just do not see the concept of a "paradigm" as having any functional use in describing major shifts in gerontology—as gerontology does not fit conveniently into any single disciplinary mold—nor can we apply the conditions of Kuhnian revolutionary science and paradigmatic shifts to the study of ageing.

We understand that it is a matter of debate to consider the use of paradigm versus inflection points, and it is the subject of further debate to consider *five inflection points* over a span of time (see Table 3.1), but we believe it will be even more contentious for some readers to consider that a new inflection point [5.0] will become the new prevailing theme in gerontology beyond the proposed and current one labeled as *Optimal Ageing* [4.0]).

To reinterpret the developments and shifts in gerontology from an historical perspective (in hindsight) by using inflection points is one thing, but to offer a prospective prevailing theme (such as [5.0]) before any critical mass has taken

And so the price of our immortality is our humanity.~ Nick Lane (2009). *Life Ascending: The Ten Great Inventions of Evolution*, W.W. Norton & Co. p. 285.

K.F. Felsted and S.D. Wright, *Toward Post Ageing*,
Healthy Ageing and Longevity 1, DOI 10.1007/978-3-319-09051-1_3

Table 3.1 Inflection Points

(Directional Shifts in Prevailing Theme in gerontology/ageing)
[1.0]: Philosophy of Ageing (ageing as *reflection*)
[2.0]: Bio-medical Diseases of Ageing (ageing as a *problem*)
[3.0]: Demographics of Ageing (ageing as a *challenge*)
Proposed current theme:
[4.0]: Optimal Ageing (ageing as a *reward*)
Proposed emergent theme:
[5.0]: Post Ageing (ageing as an *artifact*)

place to verify and corroborate the theme actually exists is bound to be a risky venture, a conjecture, even an adventure. But such is the purpose of this book: to tread carefully, but with courage and integrity, so as to look ahead and create the profile for what we think is the next inflection point in gerontological research, teaching, and application. Having said that, we want to remind the reader that the inflection point structure does not imply that each new and emerging "prevailing theme-to-be" does not simply replace the contributions and perspectives of the previous prevailing theme in gerontology (contra the Kuhnian notion of "paradigms")—nor do we claim any sort of incommensurability between inflection points. As we have stated before, it is assumed that the previous themes are very much still active (to one degree or another) in gerontology and have their functional place in the literature, but the dynamics in the study of ageing are such that some themes (and sub-themes) emerge and prevail and then reach of point of stasis (and in some cases stagnation) in research, in the pedagogical currency of the classroom, and in the field as application and "practice." More often than not, the stasis profile (which is characterized by little or no change in the direction or momentum of the scholarship) is very close to what Thomas Kuhn did come to recognize as "normal science" (or "puzzle-solving"), such that "the field" drifts along—quite content to follow the prevailing lodestar that is the overarching raison d'être for where it is headed. And currently, it is proposed that the prevailing theme and majority of "action" in gerontology is now supporting and advocating for *optimal ageing*.

In this case, it matters little at the meta-theoretical level of the field (or from the aerial viewpoint or bird's-eye view) that we in gerontology ponder the nuances of modernism or post-modernism, or the use of quantitative or qualitative methodologies, or whether or not we actually use explicit theory or not (most likely we do not); rather, the guiding *Weltanschauung* for most of us (when asked—or when we self-identify with it) is still associated with the prevailing theme (i.e., "optimal ageing" and the attending research which focuses on life satisfaction and happiness, or "subjective well-being" (SWB) which cross-cuts, weaves, and intersects into almost all that we do, both didactically and clinically. This is what we preach within the field and it serves as an encompassing vision for the entire field of study and practice—regardless of academic debates about molecular or molar theories, cross-sectional or longitudinal methods, or whether the project is funded by corporate entities or community-based grants.

But here we are at the cusp of a new inflection point that is identified as [5.0] Post Ageing (ageing as an *artifact*), and this change in direction is very much influenced by the rapid developments and advancements by what Joel Garreau (2005) refers to as a "radical evolution" in the human condition, and to a large degree what researchers such as Aubrey de Grey believe is "the end of ageing." Garreau (2005) proposes that these varied new technologies will offer both promise and peril in the enhancement of our minds, bodies, "and what it means to be human." And we, along with Garreau (2005), believe that the convergence of four inter-related, intertwining technologies—*genetic, robotic, information,* and *nano processes* (hereafter known as GRIN technologies; see Garreau 2005)—represents the new inflection point for gerontology [5.0] into the first half of this century. Although others (see Roden 2010; and see h + Magazine, Winter 2009; http://www.hplusmagazine.com) have proposed a similar (and highly related) acronym of "NBIC" which stands for *nano-bio-info-cogno* technologies, we prefer Garreau's acronym for the purposes of this book.

As the reader shall soon discover, some of the scholarship in the field of gerontology related to the use of *technologies* is theoretically being grouped into a several categories (i.e., gerotechnology, assistive technology), some of which still have connections with previous inflection points as strategies to prevent, delay, or compensate for the perceptual, cognitive, and physical declines of ageing ([2.0]) and the use of technology to support or enhance the opportunities associated with ageing ([4.0])related to communication, leisure, learning, service, and artistic expression (see Fozard et al. 2000; Hudson 2014). But because the intersect of technology and bioengineering with Ageing are seen as a critical feature to distinguish [4.0] from [5.0], we will also acknowledge that the change in direction of inflection points is not overtly dramatic and not like the assumed "switch" that would take place in some Kuhnian "paradigm shift." As the reader will discover, there are incremental developments within the inflection point change in direction, and as the curvature suggests it is a gradual process. Nevertheless, a change does take place in the prevailing view. Thus, one of our goals is to differentiate the various uses of technologies by using the inflection point heuristic in the study of ageing so that we can better understand the purposes, function, goals, and stated outcomes of the categories of technologies as they relate to the study of the ageing process and ageing condition of the individual. As a brief example of our intent with the heuristic, one can imagine that technologies used to address ageing as a *problem* will be different in purpose, function, and application when compared to Ageing as a *reward*, and then again different from the uses of technologies to transcend or move beyond the ageing process entirely (*Post Ageing*, or ageing as an *artifact*). Yet, all of the exemplars to be noted for [5.0] have technology and/or bioengineering as the center focus for ageing research, teaching precepts, and applications. Our goal with the typology will be to examine more closely the various developments within post ageing and then to assign these incremental "versions" of development a number (e.g., [5.1]; [5.2]; [5.3] and so on) to correspond with the movement and progress toward a positive curvature in the inflection point [5.0] derivative.

Despite the incremental developments, it would be easy to understand why there would be substantial resistance and skepticism by some readers to embrace the notion of *any* kind of new inflection point [5.0] for gerontology based on various budding technologies that have seemingly inundated every facet of the human condition. One reason would be that that such a focus would be interpreted as a direct assault on the existential and humanistic traditions in the study of the ageing process. In other words, the proposed [5.0] inflection point would supposedly strip away the essence of what makes us human, especially the significance as an ageing individual with spiritual and philosophical characteristics that transcend the reductionism and consilience found in the scientific domains of biology and technology (see DeLashmutt 2006). For example, Roger Scruton (2010) has creatively referred to one trend of rewriting the human person by rewiring the human brain as "neurotrash"—the attempt to reduce the "I" to the fMRI.

Another reason for incredulity when considering a new inflection point for the domain of gerontology would be the substantive lack of inclusion and coverage of the impact of these intertwining GRIN technologies (*genetic, robotic, information,* and *nano* processes; see Garreau 2005) in the majority of handbooks and encyclopedias that offer a supposed comprehensive review of theory, research, and application in the field of ageing. For example, in the second edition of the *Handbook of Theories of Ageing* (Bengtson et al. 2009) there is little presentation or discussion of the GRIN technologies, although it is understood that the handbook is primarily presenting an overview of theories and models; nevertheless, the coverage is minimal, and ironically the one time it is addressed in the handbook, it is presented in an "integrative model" for gerontology (Bass 2009). This model not only includes "technology" in the integration matrix (see "A."), but the author (Bass 2009) also uses a metaphor and graphical model that is inherently "technological"—a "radio tower structure" (see Fig. 19.1; p. 362 in Bass 2009)—in order to indicate the need for greater integration between various micro- and macro-level forces and influences on the ageing individual. Although we like the integrative model and the metaphor (the conceptual model that is evolving) that Bass (2009) has proposed, we believe it needs to be much more inclusive (to capture the dramatic developments in the GRIN technologies) in order to be a relevant and an integrative model for gerontology in this century. Part of the rationale for writing this book is the nuances of the *Post Ageing* inflection point, and it is our responsibility to further elaborate on inflection point [5.0] and the developments associated with this curvature [5.x].

But we need to continue our examination of how these technologies have been addressed thus far—starting with the larger and comprehensive handbooks and encyclopedias. In *The Cambridge Handbook of Age and Ageing*, the editors Johnson et al. (2005) have included seven parts, 72 chapters, 110 contributors, and 744 pages worth of materials. In addition to an entire section devoted to "The Ageing Body" (Part Two), there is a chapter (see pp. 662–669) on "Adaptation to *New Technologies*" by Charness and Czaja (2005), focusing attention on "contexts in which older adults will use technology and how technology, when well designed, can promote quality of life and independence for older people" (p. 662). There is also an entry for "technology" in *The Encyclopedia of Ageing* edited by Shulz et al. (2006), but again the discussion is brief.

So is the domain of gerontology completely bereft of the discussion of technology as it intersects the ageing process? Of course not (see Hudson 2014). But before we examine the specific works in the literature of the last decade it is important to review the typology proposed by Garreau (2005), which we prefer to use, in order to frame the emergent inflection point [5.0] associated with the GRIN technologies (*genetic, robotic, information,* and *nano* processes). We believe it is important to review this so we can assess the developments and applications of technologies in ageing so far—and what we in the field will need to consider in the near future, if not the immediate present.

References

Bass, S. A. (2009). Toward an integrative theory of social gerontology. In V. Bengtson, M. Silverstein, N. Putney, & D. Gans (Eds.), *Handbook of Theories of Ageing* (2nd ed., pp. 347–374). New York, NY: Springer.

Bengtson, V. L., Gans, D., Putney, N., & Silverstein, M. (2009). *Handbook of Theories of Ageing*. New York: Springer.

Charness, N., & Czaja, S. J. (2005). Adaptation to new technologies. In M. L. Johnson, V. Bengtson, P. Coleman, & T. Kirkwood (Eds.), *The Cambridge Handbook of Age and Ageing* (pp. 662–669). New York: Cambridge University Press.

DeLashmutt, M. W. (2006). A better life through information technology? The techno-theological eschatology of post human speculative science (Perspectives on techno-science and human nature). *Zygon, 41*, 267–287.

Fozard, J. L., Rietsema, J., Bouman, H., & Graafmans, A. M. (2000). Gerotechnology: Creating enabling environments for the challenges and opportunities of Ageing. *Educational Gerontology, 26*(4), 331–344.

Garreau, J. (2005). *Radical Evolution: the Promise and Peril of Enhancing Our Minds, Our Bodies—and What It Means to Be Human*. New York: Broadway Random House.

Hudson, R. B. (2014). Ageing and technology: The promise and the paradox. *Public Policy & Ageing Report, 24*, 3–5.

Johnson, M. L., Bengtson, V., Coleman, P., & Kirkwood, T. (2005). *The Cambridge Handbook of Age and Ageing*. New York: Cambridge University Press.

Roden, D. (2010). Deconstruction and excision in philosophical posthumanism. *Journal of Evolution & Technology, 21*(1), 27–36.

Scruton, R. (2010). Neurotrash. *TPM, 50*, 98–99 (Third Quarter).

Shulz, R., Noelker, L. S., Rockwood, K., & Sprott, R. L. (2006). *The Encyclopedia of Ageing* (4th ed.). New York: Springer.

Chapter 4
[5.1] to [5.2] Moderate Versions of the Inflection Point and Positive Derivative

Abstract In the discussion of the shift from [4.0] to the different versions of [5.x] inflection points, we will introduce a secondary degree typology to categorize the developments along the change in direction (and along the positive derivative) using the labels of *moderate* and *radical* regarding the intersection of technology with ageing issues. The demarcation between the two will be determined by the direct relevance to and association with the GRIN technologies (Garreau 2005), (*genetic, robotic, information,* and *nano* processes). The *moderate* versions of the [5.x] inflection point have ample connections and references to technology and Ageing in the publications and still represent the prevailing view, but the topics have primarily focused on assistive technology, the human factor, applied psychology and cognitive science (see Helal et al. 2008).The moderate versions have focused on the use of the Internet by older adults, computer-mediated and computer-based communication, household and safety monitoring, and tele-health applications (see Grierson et al. 2009; Kang et al. 2010; Orlov 2010). In order to reach the *radical* version of the emergent inflection point—and thus merit a greater inflection point "score" [5.x]—the publication would have to explicitly indicate the intersection of technologies and bioengineering issues with the Ageing process to which Garreau (2005) has alluded.

Keywords Artificial intelligence · Assistive technology · Biotechnology · Gerontechnology · Gerotechnology · Moderate version · Nanotechnology · Neuroplasticity · Radical version · Robotics

4.1 [5.1] to [5.2] Moderate Versions of the Inflection Point

As stated, we will use the year 2000 as a benchmark, both as a matter of convenience and as a preference to indicate the "turn of the century" (from a historical perspective) as we review and assess the literature thus far relating to Ageing and technologies and our proposed heuristic of inflection points.

K.F. Felsted and S.D. Wright, *Toward Post Ageing*,
Healthy Ageing and Longevity 1, DOI 10.1007/978-3-319-09051-1_4

The best place to start in the literature is with the publication, *Gerontechnology: Creating enabling environments for the challenges and opportunities of ageing*, by Fozard et al. (2000). Our decision to use the year 2000 as a breakpoint to examine the shift in direction should be qualified by the appreciation of many examples in the literature that serve as precursors to the proposed [5.0] inflection point in gerontology. While we use this article as the starting position because it offers a nice review of the literature up until that date, please note that the topic of technology's intersect with the human condition does not begin with this work. For example, we should marvel at the earlier philosophical scholarship reflections of Martin Heidegger on this topic with his publication, *The Question Concerning Technology* (which corresponds to the [1.0] curvature in our heuristic), written in 1954 (see also Hanks 2009; Olsen et al. 2009). We also would draw attention to the prescient works of Alvin Toffler with his publications *Future Shock* (1970) and *The Third Wave* (1987) (which corresponds to the [3.0] curvature in our heuristic). In an article in the *New Scientist* (1994) titled, "Alvin Toffler: still shocking after all these years: *New Scientist* meets the controversial futurologist," Toffler shared what inspired him to write *Future Shock*,

> Our ideas came together in 1965 in an article called 'The future as a way of life', which argued that change was going to accelerate and that the speed of change could induce disorientation in lots of people. We coined the phrase 'future shock' as an analogy to the concept of culture shock. With future shock you stay in one place but your own culture changes so rapidly that it has the same disorienting effect as going to another culture.

In effect, Toffler's assessment of "future shock" as a barometer of social transformation in large part due to technology advancements is an important thread that weaves into the unfolding of the [5.0] inflection point for the study of ageing and for understanding the ageing process into the 21st century.

In the discussion of the shift from [4.0] to the different versions of [5.x] inflection points, we will introduce a secondary degree typology to categorize the developments along the change in direction (and along the positive derivative) using the labels of *moderate* and *radical* regarding the intersection of technology with ageing issues. The demarcation between the two will be determined by the direct relevance to and association with the GRIN technologies (Garreau 2005), (*genetic, robotic, information,* and *nano* processes). The *moderate* versions of the [5.x] inflection point have ample connections and references to technology and ageing in the publications and still represent the prevailing view, but the topics have primarily focused on assistive technology, the human factor, applied psychology and cognitive science (see Helal et al. 2008).The moderate versions have focused on the use of the Internet by older adults, computer-mediated and computer-based communication, household and safety monitoring, and tele-health applications (see Grierson et al. 2009; Kang et al. 2010; Orlov 2010). In order to reach the *radical* version of the emergent inflection point—and thus merit a greater inflection point "score" [5.x]—the publication would have to explicitly indicate the intersection of technologies and bioengineering issues with the ageing process to which Garreau (2005) has alluded.

Now, back to the publication, *Gerontechnology: Creating enabling environments for the challenges and opportunities of ageing,* where the authors (Fozard et al. 2000) offered an overview of the "new discipline" of gerotechnology and described the special needs and interests of older persons with respect to technology in six areas: (a) housing, (b) communication (see another publication: *Communication, Technology and Ageing, Opportunities and Challenges for the Future* by Charness et al. 2000, on this topic), (c) personal mobility and transportation, (d) health, (e) work, and (f) recreation and self-fulfillment. Notably the authors defined *gerontechnology* as "engineering and technology for the benefit of ageing and aged people" (p. 332) and they indicated that the term *gerontechnology* was actually coined by Graafsman and Brouwers in 1989. Based on the heuristic previously discussed, this article has the connections with two previous inflection points: [2.0] and [4.0]; that is, Fozard et al. (2000) indicated how engineering and technologies can either assist (thus, *assistive technology*) in compensating for losses with ageing process, or delay, or even prevent them ([2.0]). Fozard et al. (2000 then indicated how these same engineering changes could facilitate opportunities for older adults "by enhancing technical application for daily living, communication, transportation, safe workplaces, learning, and artistic endeavors" (p. 332; [4.0]). But when using the GRIN technologies typology (*genetic, robotic, information,* and *nano* processes, see Garreau 2005), this publication does not quite capture the essence of the latter developments (*radical* version) but is acknowledged as a change in direction of a prevailing view under the aegis of "post ageing", and so this publication merits a *moderate* version [5.1] inflection point.

The next publication we highlight is *Impact of Technology on Successful Ageing*, edited by Charness and Schaie (2003), which provided a detailed examination of changes in technology that impact individuals as they age with an emphasis upon cultural contexts and person-environment fit from human factors, from psychological and sociological perspectives. Charness and Schaie (2003) take into consideration the role of macro-influences in shaping technological changes in industrialized societies affecting successful ageing in terms of quality of life. Out of several topics discussed, there is an emphasis on human factors and ageing, the impact of the Internet, and assistive technology. Given the array of chapters and topics addressed, the publication edited by Charness and Schaie (2003) has connections to at least three previous inflection points based on our proposed heuristic: [2.0]—Ageing as a *problem*; [3.0]—Ageing as a *challenge*; [4.0]—Ageing as a *reward*, but again we do not think that this publication necessarily presents the *radical* version of technology. It does represent a change in direction associated with the sprouting inflection point [5.0] toward post ageing and so this publication merits a [5.1] inflection point, a moderate version.

The same analysis and interpretation, meriting a [5.1] inflection point, can be applied to the next publication, *Technology for Adaptive Ageing* (Pew and Van Hemel 2004) which is the product of a workshop designed to identify high payoff areas in the technological devices that assist people ageing normally, as well as those with disabilities and impairments (see also Helal et al. 2008). There were also six areas examined in this publication: communication, employment, health, learning, living environments, and transportation. Again, while there is ample discussion of the intersect of technology with the ageing process, the level of inflection point focus is on ageing as *problem*, *challenge*, or *reward*, which reflect the previous inflection points [2.0], [3.0], and [4.0] and thus represents the [5.1] moderate version along the curvature.

The next publication to be discussed, *Gerotechnology: Research and Practice in Technology and Ageing* (Burdick and Kwon 2004), is interpreted as a slightly stronger (but still moderate version, thus [5.2], of the post ageing exemplar associated with the positive derivative. This book extends the agenda of previous inflection points where technology (or gerotechnology) is promoted as having as its main purpose and function building connections to the previous prevailing viewpoints of ageing as a *problem*, as a *challenge*, and as a *reward*. Such an interpretation is validated by the review of books and the resulting interpretation published by Russell Morgan (2005) in *The Gerontologist* (pp. 704–710), with the eye-catching title of "Technology Greets the Age Wave." The three books that Morgan reviewed were previously mentioned in this work (*Gerotechnology: Research and Practice in Technology and Ageing*, Burdick and Kwon, 2004; *Impact of Technology on Successful Ageing,* Charness and Schaie 2003; and *Technology for Adaptive Ageing*, Pew and Van Hemel 2004).

Gerotechnology: Research and Practice in Technology and Ageing (Burdick and Kwon 2004) is an edited book and so the topics are varied and comprehensive—Section B (Computers, Older Adults, and Caregivers), Section C (Assistive technology in the Home and Environment), and Section D (Models, Prototypes and Specific Applications)—offering, for the most part, the traditional perspectives (i.e., moderate) on the intersect of ageing and technology. Three specific chapters represent the various levels (or versions of the [5.x] inflection point) as far as extending the scientific conversation relating to the [5.0] inflection point. First, a chapter (which is actually the epilogue) by Fozard (2004), titled "Applications to Ageing Are Helping Human Factors and Ergonomics To Grow Up Right" that we found inadequate. "Inadequate" in the sense that the edited book had no sense of "looking forward" to what possible developments could (or should) occur. Instead, the epilogue focused on the specific domain of gerotechnology that related to human factors and ergonomics (which, granted, is an important aspect of the domain), but it has the limited perspective of a historical reflection. We found this to be disappointing because it promoted and then highlighted a specific dimension of what gerotechnology could embrace and include but neglected to entertain any discussions or applications of the radical versions of the inflection point as it related to the emergence of GRIN technologies.

Another chapter is titled, "Ageing and Technology—Social Science Approaches" by Mollenkopf (2004). We found this to be one-dimensional in the sense that, while it was the prerogative of the author to emphasize a "social science perspective" (over, let's say, a bio-technological one), it is nevertheless concerning that the author claimed to be interested in the balance of "micro-levels approaches" (previous research related to human factors and ergonomics) (p. 56) which is assumed to be the prevailing approach with gerotechnology—the so-called "macro-conditions" of socio-cultural contexts of symbolism and "cultural and action theory" (p. 64).The author seems to believe that the "socio-constructivist" approach could have had more to say on the intersection of technology and ageing, but evidently failed to deliver on that promise and potential. The irony of all this retrospection and review by Mollenkopf (2004) on the macro-conditions for technology and ageing is that while the author proceeded to then call for "integrating technology into a holistic, integrated approach" (p. 56), we felt that the author may actually have missed the mark. Mollenkopf announced that,

> …social science technology perspectives seem to offer the most suitable framework for linking and integrating the most important micro and macro aspects of human Ageing and social and technological change in a larger societal and historical view (p. 64).

We must respond, in that while the social science perspectives may have the most to say (which is their prerogative) about larger societal and historical perspectives, we do not think that it is then necessarily "the most suitable framework for linking micro and macro aspects." Based on this chapter in the book, we failed to find any solid evidence that these specific social perspectives were "holistic" or "integrated" or even representative of micro-macro linkages. In our opinion, they are simply more of the same macro level (theoretical) perspectives that have dominated the (heretofore) moderate versions of this inflection point. The focus (with the moderate version) has been on environmental and contextual factors that interact with the human activities, but there is little to be found in these perspectives that address the burgeoning field of the GRIN technologies that often reflect more of the biological, cognitive, genetic, and the neurosciences. Our point is this: in order to truly grasp the "micro" levels that area part of the technology and ageing intersect, Mollenkopf (2004) and others will have to extend their "holistic" vision beyond the human factors and ergonomic dimensions as the supposed end-point of the micro-level approach. With the advent of GRIN technologies and their intersect with the ageing condition, a truly "holistic", integrated approach will have to include the radical versions of this domain of technology and ageing. While it is perfectly acceptable have to have macro level theories and perspectives in the integrated and holistic models, it would be extremely limited and short-sighted to not incorporate the emergent radical versions that are more micro. We will discuss the *more micro* issues later in this book, but to illustrate our point here, we think it imperative for gerontology to understand technology not just as "something out there" interacting with ageing individuals in order to assist in their activities of daily living (ADLs or IADLs), but as having a "nature" that can evolve and transform itself over time (Arthur 2009). Furthermore, to solely rely upon the social sciences as the most suitable framework to understand the complete range, the full scale of technologies, that affect and influence the ageing process will potentially overlook the emergent perspectives in psychology, biotechnology, brain plasticity, linguistics, neuroscience, nanotechnology, nanomedicine, artificial intelligence, robotics, and human-computer systems that reflect the "embodied mind" and "cognitive extension" perspectives (Chodzko-Zajko et al. 2009; Clark 2010;

Gazzaniga 2008; Hanna and Maiese 2009; Jones 2004; Lakoff and Johnson 1999; Read et al. 2008) that should *complement* the macro-level perspectives in any "gerotechnology" (or "gerontechnology").

The last chapter to discuss in the edited book, *Gerotechnology: Research and Practice in Technology and Ageing* by Burdick and Kwon (2004), is entitled "Ethical Realities: The Old, the New, and the Virtual" and is authored by Gari Lesnoff-Caravaglia (2004). We think it is the strongest (more of a *radical* version than the other *moderate* chapters) and most forward thinking of all the chapters in the book. This wide-ranging chapter anchors the examination of gerotechnology in both a historical perspective (Lesnoff-Caravaglia makes connections to previous inflection point themes, such as discussing the role of technology in the philosophical works of Heidegger, previously mentioned in this section) as well as a prospective vision—especially in the context of ethical issues. For example, Lesnoff-Caravaglia (2004) stated the reciprocal relationship between technology and ageing in this fashion:

> The societal effects of technological change and the Ageing of the population are likely to be felt in various ways: health status, living environments, and work. The creation, dissemination and use of technology involves not only mastery of sciences and engineering tools and concepts, but the ability to cope with a difficult set of ethical and economic issues and choices (p. 245).

And in this edited book, we were surprised and pleased to see—at long last—a commentary about the future in terms of expanded and more elaborate uses of technology,

> In the near future there may well be an increased fusion of the biological and the technological. It is already predicted that the majority of surgical procedures in the future will be on the order of organ transplants and the implanting of a variety of prostheses. The goal of such prostheses may include the *enhancement* or ameliorization of sensory functions such as vision and hearing *beyond what are currently considered normal capabilities.* Night vision, distance hearing, and specialized gloves for tactile discrimination are increasingly part of the technological armamentarium (p. 248; emphasis added).

As evidenced in the excerpt above, Lesnoff-Caravaglia (2004) has touched upon the very nature of the radical versions of technology that are part of the landscape addressed by Garreau with the GRIN technologies (see also Lesnoff-Caravaglia 2007). We found Lesnoff-Caravaglia's chapter to be deeply philosophical in the sense that accurate and relevant questions were posed concerning the ethical issues surrounding the use of technologies in relation to the implications of potential scientific breakthroughs that focus on the "problem" of ageing (see also, Bramstedt 2001; Hackler 2001). The reader senses that while Lesnoff-Caravaglia had one foot well-grounded in the traditions of the past, she also felt comfortable recognizing and embracing the inevitable changes that lay ahead with the evolution of technology. Interestingly enough, Lesnoff-Caravaglia (2004) was able to make the conceptual connection of how both technology and the study of ageing have much in common in terms of structure and content; thus, we found the following statement (in the excerpt below) to be the quintessential description of the [5.0] inflection point—and one that captures the developments along the curvature of the positive derivative from a moderate version [5.1, 5.2] to more radical versions [5.3, 5.4, 5.5…5.x],

> Technology and ageing are very similar in one respect—they both have an onward or forward movement. There is no going back. Once a technology is invented and proves to be useful, it is changed only to become even more complex and does not disappear. Ageing also moves forward in an inexorable fashion. In this sense, technology and ageing are both structured by time (p. 254).

Before we indicate the three publications that best represent the transition from the *moderate* [5.1, 5.2] to the *radical* version of the inflection point/curvature [5.3, 5.4] we will conduct a partial inventory of the burgeoning amount of literature that has emerged to represent the *moderate* version of the [5.x] inflection point.

4.2 [5.1] to [5.2]: Additional Moderate Versions of the Inflection Point and Positive Derivative—Further Examples Indicating the Curvature

Our goal here is to illustrate examples along the 5.1 and 5.2 curvatures, which represent the traditional domains of gerotechnology and assistive technology. The issue of *Science Studies* (Volume 17, No. 2, 2004) with guest editor Britt Östlund examined the intersection of ageing and technology using primarily a social constructivist (socio-technical) perspective. Utilizing a similar approach were the publications by Agree et al. (2004) who examined the factors influencing the use of mobility technology in community-based long-term care and Lansley et al. (2004) who studied the use and adaptations of assistive technology enabling older people to remain in their homes. Mann (2005) edited the book *Smart Technology for Ageing, Disability, and Independence—The State of the Science,* which presented a comprehensive look at "smart technology" for home and community including the various uses of assistive technology and robotics. Cutler (2005) provided a nice overview of the connection between ageism and technology (noting a reciprocal influence), and then there was the special issue of *Generations,* Summer 2006 with Czaja and Schulz (2006) as guest editors, offering a nice cross-section of articles relating to the moderate version of the inflection point and curvature. Sara Czaja continues her scholarship in this track with a significant co-authored publication (Czaja et al. 2006) titled, "Factors Predicting the Use of Technology: Findings from the Center for Research and Education on Ageing and Technology Enhancement (CREATE)" in the journal *Psychology and Ageing.* This article by Czaja et al. (2006) is categorized and definitively placed in the moderate version with its focus on the successful adoption of technology (primarily the use of computers and the Internet) as an important factor to increase functional independence in community-dwelling adults (see also Hammel 2000). In the *Journal of Housing for the Elderly*, Mahmood et al. (2008) discussed a pilot project exploring attitudes, opinions, and preferences of older adults concerning the use of technology to support and extend their ability to "age in place". Readers should also refer to the web site publication of the American Association of Homes and Services for the Ageing (http://www.aahsa.org) to view a complete report on the "State of Technology in Ageing Services."

In other examples of the moderate version of post ageing [5.1, 5.2], Weiner et al. (2003) described the uses of information technology to improve the health care of older adults; Skubic et al. (2009) discussed the role of passive sensor networks used for monitoring older adults in their homes, and Steel and Gray (2009) reviewed the published studies to describe issues surrounding assistive technology (AT) use by baby boomers (see also Lindenberger 2008). Clarke et al. (2009) examined the demographic and social characteristics of mobility device (assistive technology) users in long-term settings, and Topo and Östlund (2009) examined the uses of technology to better meet the needs of people of dementia. Kitchener et al. (2008) analyzed data related to assistive technology in Medicaid Home-and Community-Based Waiver Programs (see also Resnik and Allen 2006). In a track related to the use of technological devices by older adults, Slegers et al. (2009) examined the role of cognitive functional decline, whereas Wright and Hill (2009) stated concerns about the over-reliance of Internet access for older adults to a obtain information about Medicare part D, with concerns that both issues of increased disability as well as decreased income would affect computer/internet access for many older adults—thereby increasing the stratification of access to health care (see also Charness and Boot 2009). But Godfrey and Johnson (2009) offer potential solutions to these classification challenges by describing the role of informal networks ("digital circles of support", many of them older adults who are "technology literate mediators") in assisting other older adults, facilitating both groups as engaged citizens in their own care. Lai (2008) examined the use of information and communication technologies (ICT) and its effects on inter-generational dynamics in Japan, while Hernandez-Encuentra et al. (2009) examined the topic in Spain. Finally, it should be noted that the International Society for Gerontechnology (ISG) represents a professional organization capturing the spirit of the moderate version of the curvature—which has as its mission:

> ISG encourages and promotes technological innovations in products and services that address older peoples' ambitions and needs on the basis of scientific knowledge about ageing processes including cultural and individual differences (http://gerontechnology.info/index.php/journal/pages/view/journal).

Further, the aim of the journal publication is:

> to provide a forum for reporting original research, review papers, and personal perspectives on the broad area of fitting technological environments to support changing life goals and lifestyle preferences into advanced age. Research outcomes reported in the Journal form the basis—for designers, architects, standards developers, builders, engineers, marketers, manufacturers, medical doctors, pharmacists, decision makers, and related professionals in the health, social, business and technology professions—to provide the proper environment for the greatest number of people in society.

Readers are encouraged to visit the website for the Center for Aging Services Technologies (CAST) (www.leadingage.org/cast.aspx) which focuses on the development, evaluation, and adoption of emerging technologies that improve the ageing experience. These technologies were highlighted in several *New York Times* newspaper articles (July 29, 2010) that related to the use of technologies for ageing in place (see Taub 2010, "The Technology for Monitoring Elderly Relatives") and in the publication by Kang et al. (2010) in the *Journal of American Geriatrics Society* as well as the Public Policy Report and Ageing Report, Volume 24 (see Hudson 2014).

But before we move into the transition exemplars for [5.3] and [5.4], we propose that the article by Joyce and Loe (2009) offer several important implications for the consideration of differentiations within post ageing ([5.x] in general). In their article, "A Sociological Approach to Ageing, Technology and Health," Joyce and Loe (2009) raise provocative questions about the role of older adults (as the consumers), the biomedicalization of ageing, and the rise of gerontechnology industries and professions to better understand health and illness. In essence, Joyce and Loe (2009) call for a new approach that puts "elders' meaning making, creativity, and bodies at the centre of analysis of technology, science, and health" (p. 172). In other words, older adults are to be viewed as knowledgeable techno-scientific users rather than as victims of technology and design. Furthermore, Joyce and Loe (2009) propose an intriguing demarcation between assistive technologies and anti-ageing medicine. On one side of the technology and ageing intersect (thus post ageing), is the field of anti-ageing medicine which is purported to be an extension of biomedicalization processes and where the ageing process is seen as "pathological"—as something to be overcome—and youthfulness is to be restored (as a result of biotechnological intervention) as the desired state of existence. On the other side of the intersect are the assistive technologies which are purported to empower the older adult to age in place via "transforming technologies and inclusive design projects" that help older adults adapt and accommodate to potential changes in various physical and cognitive abilities. The critical line drawn for the demarcation between the two domains relates to more of a philosophical approach to the ageing individual; that is, the difference is where the transformation takes place and to what purpose and outcome. Joyce and Loe (2009) appear to take exception to the notion that the ageing process is understood by advocates within anti-ageing medicine as pathology, whereas from the gerontechnology perspective, "the ageing body is still enabled and constrained, but it is not targeted for transformation from the inside out as it is in anti-ageing medicine" (p. 174). So here we see the key demarcation indicators according to Joyce and Loe (2009) as that which either transforms the external environment (gerontechnology) or the internal (physiological) environment (anti-ageing); supposedly seeking internal transformations is thus seen as reflecting "ageist" tendencies because of the position that "youthful bodies" are the norm (the ageing body is not a given) whereas with external transformations, the older adult maintains dignity and agentic capabilities, while embracing the ageing experience (senescence) as normal and natural. In our opinion, such demarcations are useful in stimulating discussion and dialogue, but also raise further questions in regards to the validity of making such a distinction between external and internal transformations as the key element to then determine if something is "anti-ageing" or not. For example, one has to wonder how hearing aids may be that different from a prosthetic device or the implantation of artificial devices that replace bones, organs or tissues. Perhaps it is the introduction of robotics, or artificial intelligence, or bioengineering or some other variable that is the key element to help clarify—but Joyce and Loe (2009) did not address this any further. Here is one example that indicates our point about demarcations representing an interesting radical application of technologies, yet remaining external to the ageing individual. Nejat et al. (2010) have proposed the use of assistive robots into the health sector, particularly in resident care practice in long-term care nursing facilities. The use of assistive robots represents a high end use of technologies such as sensory and artificial intelligence that surpasses the technology of hearing aids, yet the resident-robot interaction represents two distinct spheres (dyadic, not integrated). This is in contrast to the notion of weaving cyborg technologies internal to the human organism as a mechanism to offset the consequences of ageing. The use of assistive robots in health care applications assumes the ageing process as a given in the human organism, but offers robotic technology as supplement to social care and monitoring strategies for the older adult in long term care facilities. The work by Nejat et al. (2010) is extremely inventive and no doubt a strong candidate for the transition to radical post ageing, but includes little discussion about the ethical issues involved with robots as supplementary—or even complementary—to human staffing in long term facilities. Some may argue this represents an abdication of the care ethic for older adults in our society, while others may see this as a necessary strategy for meeting the shortage challenges in nursing staff as well as the high rate of turnover in nursing assistants. We revisit these issues in the last section of this book when we address post ageing in the context of philosophical issues.

References

Agree, E., Freedman, V., & Sengupta, M. (2004). Factors influencing the use of mobility technology in community-based long-term care. *Journal of Ageing and Health, 16*(2), 267–307.

Arthur, W. B. (2009). *The nature of technology—what it is and how evolves*. New York: Free Press.

Bramstedt, K. (2001). Scientific breakthroughs: Cause or cure of the Ageing 'problem'. *Gerontology, 47*, 52–54.

Burdick, D. C., & Kwon, S. (2004). *Gerotechnology: Research and practice in technology and Ageing*. Springfield: Charles C. Thomas Publishers.

Charness, N., & Boot, W. R. (2009). Ageing and information technology use: Potential and barriers. *Current Directions in Psychological Science, 18*(5), 253–258.

Charness, N., & Schaie, K. W. (Eds.). (2003). *Impact of technology on successful Ageing*. New York: Springer Publishing Company.

Charness, N., Park, D., & Sabel, B. (Eds.). (2000). *Communication, technology, and Ageing. Opportunities and challenges for the future*. New York: Springer.

Chodzko-Zajko, W., Kramer, A. K., & Poon, L. W. (2009). *Enhancing cognitive functioning and brain plasticity*. Champaign: Human Kinetics Publishers.

Clark, A. (2010). *Supersizing the mind: Embodiment, action, and cognitive extension (philosophy of the mind)*. New York: Oxford University Press.

Clarke, P., Chan, P., Santaguida, P., & Colantonio, A. (2009). The use of mobility devices among institutionalized older adults. *Journal of Ageing and Health, 21*(4), 611–626.

Cutler, S. (2005). Ageism and technology. *Generations, 23*(3), 67–72.

Czaja, S. J., & Schulz, R (Guest Eds.). (2006). Innovations in technology and Ageing (Introduction). *Generations, 30*(2), 6–8 (Summer).

Czaja, S. J., Charness, N., Fisk, A., Hertzog, C., Rogers, W., Nari, S., et al. (2006). Factors predicting the use of technology: Findings from the center for research and education on Ageing and technology enhancement (CREATE). *Psychology and Ageing, 21*(2), 333–352.

Fozard, J. L. (2004). Applications to Ageing are helping human factors and ergonomics to grow up right. In D. C. Burdick & S. Kwon (Eds.), *Gerotechnology: Research and practice in technology and Ageing*. Springfield: Charles C. Thomas Publishers.

Fozard, J. L., Rietsema, J., Bouman, H., & Graafmans, A. M. (2000). Gerotechnology: Creating enabling environments for the challenges and opportunities of Ageing. *Educational Gerontology, 26*(4), 331–344.

Garreau, J. (2005). *Radical evolution: The promise and peril of enhancing our minds, our bodies—and what it means to be human*. New York: Broadway Random House.

Gazzaniga, M. S. (2008). *Human: The science of what makes us unique*. New York: Ecco Books, Harper Collins.

Godfrey, M., & Johnson, O. (2009). Digital circles of support: meeting the information needs of older people. *Computers in Human Behavior, 25*, 633–642.

Grierson, L., Zelek, J., & Carnahan, H. (2009). The application of a tactile way-finding belt to facilitate navigation in older persons. *Ageing International, 34*(4), 203–215.

Hackler, C. (2001). Troubling implications of doubling the human lifespan. *Generations, 25*(Winter 2001–2002), 15–19.

Hammel, J. (2000). Assistive technology and environmental intervention (AT_EI) impact on the activity and life roles of Ageing adults with developmental disabilities. *Physical and Occupational Therapy in Geriatrics, 18*(1), 37–58.

Hanks, C. (Ed.). (2009). *Technology and values: Essential readings*. New York: Wiley-Blackwell.

Helal, A., Mokhtari, M., & Abdulrazak, B. (2008). *The engineering handbook of smart technology for Ageing, disability and independence*. Hoboken: Wiley.

Hernandez-Encuentra, E., Pousada, M., & Gomez-Zuniga, B. (2009). ICT and older people: Beyond usability. *Educational Gerontology, 35*, 226–245.

Hudson, R. B. (2014). Ageing and technology: The promise and the paradox. *Public Policy and Ageing Report, 24*, 3–5.

Jones, R. (2004). *Soft machines: Nanotechnology and life*. New York: Oxford University Press.

Joyce, K., & Loe, M. (2009). A sociological approach to ageing, technology and health. *Sociology of Health and Illness, 32*(2), 171–180.

Kang, H. (2010). In situ monitoring of health in older adults: Technologies and issues. *Journal of the American Geriatrics Society*. Retrieved July 14, 2010. doi:10.1111/j.1532-5415.2010.02959.x.

Kitchener, M., Ng, T., Lee, H., & Harrington, C. (2008). Assistive technology in Medicaid home-and community-based waiver programs. *The Gerontologist, 48*(2), 181–189.

Lai, O. (2008). The enigma of Japanese ageing-in-place practice in the information age: Does digital gadget help the (good) practice for inter-generation care? *Ageing International, 32*, 236–255.

Lakoff, G., & Johnson, M. (1999). *Philosophy in the flesh: The embodied mind and its challenge to western thought*. New York: Basic Books (Perseus Book Groups).

Lansley, P., McCreadie, C., & Tinker, A. (2004). Can adapting the homes of older people and providing assistive technology pay its way? *Age and Ageing, 33*, 571–576.

Lesnoff-Caravaglia, G. (2004). Ethical realities: The old, the new, and the virtual. In D. C. Burdick & S. Kwon (Eds.), *Gerontechnology: Growing old in a technological society*. Springfield: Charles C. Thomas Publishers.

Lesnoff-Caravaglia, G. (2007). *Gerontechnology: Growing old in a technological society*. Springfield: Charles C. Thomas Publishers.

Lindenberger, U., Lövden, M., Schellenbach, M., Li, S., & Krüger, A. (2008). Psychological principles of successful Ageing technologies: A mini-review. *Gerontology, 54*, 59–68.

Mahmood, A., Yamamoto, T., Lee, M., & Steggell, C. (2008). Perceptions and use of gerotechnology: Implications for Ageing in place. *Journal of Housing for the Elderly, 22*, 104–126.

Mann, W. (2005). *Smart technology for Ageing, disability, and independence—the state of the science*. Hoboken: Wiley.

Mollenkopf, H. (2004). Ageing and technology—social science approaches. In D. C. Burdick & S. Kwon (Eds.), *Gerotechnology: Research and practice in technology and Ageing*. Springfield: Charles C. Thomas Publishers.

Morgan, R. E. (2005). Technology meets the age wave. *The Gerontologist, 45*(2), 704–710.

Nejat, G., Nies, M., & Sexton, T. R. (2010). An interdisciplinary team for the design and integration of assistive robots in health care applications. *Home Health Care Management and Practice, 22*(2), 104–110.

New Scientist. (1994). Alvin Toffler: Still shocking after all these years. http://www.newscientist.com/article/mg14119173.500-alvin-toffler-still-shocking-after-all-these-years.html?full=true

Olsen, J. K. B., Selinger, E., & Riis, S. (2009). *New waves in philosophy of technology*. New York: Palgrave Macmillan.

Orlov, L. (2010). *Technology for Ageing in place: 2010 market overview*. http://www.ageinplacetech.com

Pew, R. W., & Van Hemel, S. B. (2004). *Technology for adaptive society*. Washington: The National Academies Press.

Read, C. Y., Green, R. C., & Smyer, M. A. (Eds.). (2008). *Ageing, biotechnology, and the future*. Baltimore: The Johns Hopkins University Press.

Resnik, L., & Allen, S. (2006). Racial and ethnic differences in use of assistive devices for mobility: Effect modification by age. *Journal of Ageing and Health, 18*(1), 106–124.

Skubic, M., Alexander, G., Popescu, M., Rantz, M., & Keller, J. (2009). A smart home application to eldercare: Current status and lessons learned. *Technology and Health Care, 17*(3), 183–201.

Slegers, K., Boxtel, M., & Jolles, J. (2009). The efficiency of using everyday technological devices by older adults: The role of cognitive functions. *Ageing and Society, 29*, 309–325.

Steel, D. M., & Gray, M. A. (2009). Baby boomers' use and perception of recommended assistive technology: A systematic review. *Disability and Rehabilitation: Assistive Technology, 4*(3), 129–136.

Taub, E. (2010). The technology for monitoring elderly relatives. *New York Times*, Retrieved July 29, 2010, from http://www.nytimes.com/2010/07/29/garden/29hometech.html

Toffler, A. (1970). *Future shock*. New York: Random House.

Toffler, A. (1987). *The third wave*. New York: Random House Value Publishing.

Topo, P., & Östlund, B. (2009). *Dementia, design and technology*. Amsterdam: IOS Press.

Weiner, M. (2003). Using information technology to improve the health care of older adults. *Annals of Internal Medicine, 139*(5, Part 2), 430–436.

Wright, D., & Hill, T. (2009). Prescription trouble: Medicare part D and patterns of computer and internet access among the elderly. *Journal of Ageing and Social Policy, 21*, 172–186.

Chapter 5
[5.3] to [5.4] Transition Publications from the *Moderate* Version of the Inflection Point (and Positive Derivative) to the *Radical* Version

Abstract The issues of ethics, morality, limits, purpose, meaning, significance, and the process of science bring us to the crossroads where the *moderate* version [5.1 to 5.4] of the inflection point will cross over to the *radical* version [5.5 and >] of the curvature and towards the activities and literature that will propel the movement onward to Post Ageing (ageing as an *artifact*). But the crossing over is not a simple bridge or even necessarily a smooth transition. Furthermore, we do not want to leave the reader with the impression that there is necessarily a demarcation between the moderate and radical versions of the curvature; rather, the incremental points ([5.1], [5.2], [5.3], [5.4] and so on) noted in the literature represent significant precursors or "portals" toward the radical version and not just a separate category of technology and ageing issues.

Keywords Ageing ethics · Ageing morality · Ageing science · Anti-ageing technologies · Ethical technology · Genetic testing · Genomics · Moderate version · Posthumanist movement · Radical version · Transhumanist movement

As mentioned earlier, we believe there are three significant publications that represent bridge, or transition, publications from the moderate version to the radical version of the positive curvature of literature representing the inflection point [5.0]. The first publication we have designated as [5.3] to indicate a continuation of the moderate version yet simultaneously an example of scholarship that is forward-looking to the radical version in terms of discussion and concrete examples. The first exemplar is associated with the journal article, "Intelligent Technology for an Ageing Population: The Use of AI to Assist Elders with Cognitive Impairment" by Pollack (2005), published in *AI Magazine,* the official publication of the Association for the Advancement of Artificial Intelligence (www.aaai.org). Pollack (2005) surveyed new technologies that incorporate artificial intelligence (AI) techniques to support older adults and help them cope with the changes of ageing, in particular cognitive decline, and also discussed the use of *robotics* (thus touching the GRIN technology threshold of Garreau 2005) in the lives of older adults (see also Nejat et al. 2010).

K.F. Felsted and S.D. Wright, *Toward Post Ageing*,
Healthy Ageing and Longevity 1, DOI 10.1007/978-3-319-09051-1_5

The second exemplar, also designated as [5.3], is represented by the book, *Gerontechnology*: *Growing Old in a Technological Society*, edited by Gari Lesnoff-Caravaglia (2007a), which offers six sections, and we believe the two chapters in Part I both represent an outstanding overview of the multi-faceted convergence of technology and ageing. It is in Part 1, Chap. 2, "Gerontechnology: The Challenge", where Lesnoff-Caravaglia (2007b) proposes an interesting and viable distinction of the uses of technology (high and low) intersecting with ageing issues. This complements our use of the heuristic for the [5.0] inflection point and the differentiation of *moderate* (low technology) and *radical* (high technology) versions of the curvature for post ageing. Lesnoff-Caravaglia (2007b) marks the distinction in this manner,

> The practical application of science can be either at the level of high technology or low technology. On occasion, simple solutions on the level of low technology, such as redesigning tools or altering home environments, have more practical outcomes. Some high technology streams such as genetics, robotics, informatics, and in particular, communication technology provide the potential for very powerful and controversial applications. For example, the science of genetics is leading to the possibility of predicting such conditions as heart disease and Alzheimer's Disease. (p. 23)

For the most part, the remaining chapters address some artificial intelligence and robotics issues, but there is less discussion on genomics and nanotechnology (using the GRIN technology template of Garreau 2005). The last chapter, "Gerontechnological Ontology: Human Experience within Extraordinary Frameworks", is especially intriguing as Lesnoff-Caravaglia analyzes the *human experience* from the perspective of the extraordinary framework for living in an ageing society. This is reminiscent of her earlier work (Lesnoff-Caravaglia 2004) in the edited book by Burdick and Kwon (2004). We found this chapter a much-needed philosophical reflection regarding the ethical and existential issues that permeate the intersection of technology with gerontology (and similar to Joyce and Loe 2009). It also may remind the reader of the cross-threads with other inflection points (i.e., ageing as a *reflection*) that still are relevant in our current prevailing theme [4.0] Optimal Ageing and the new emergent curvature of [5.x] Post Ageing. Nevertheless, the recent work of Lesnoff-Caravaglia (2007a) is indicative of the transition literature [5.3] that is developing along the post ageing curvature and her summary statement in the last chapter is insightful and prescient, "In the near future there will be an increased fusion of the biological and the technological." (p. 302)

The next publication, *Ageing, Biotechnology and the Future*, edited by Read et al. (2008), represents a further and extended transition [5.3, 5.4] to the radical version [5.5 and >] because of the heavy emphasis on *biotechnology* which is more radical (or "high technology" according to Lesnoff-Caravaglia 2007b) than the prevailing emphasis within the moderate version that primarily reflects ergonomics and assistive technology (or "low technology" according to Lesnoff-Caravaglia 2007b). So we have classified this publication by Read et al. (2008) as [5.4] on the curvature. We also found this publication to be far more advanced along the curvature, than other exemplars with [5.x] so far, due to its coverage and discussion of the GRIN technologies (Garreau 2005) with wide-ranging multidisciplinary perspectives that offered both arguments for advancing the development of biotechnologies, and in addition, constructive criticisms that need further dialogue and resolution. For example, in the Preface, the editors (Read et al. 2008) review the ethical issues that arise at the intersection of collective ageing, personal ageing, and biotechnological advances,

> Recent advances in biotechnology and our newfound understanding of the human genome have opened a door to exciting new possibilities for improving the quality and duration of life, albeit with many caveats. The idea of replacing ailing organs or tissues with healthy ones created from stem cells is gaining widespread acceptance, yet the use of related technology to reproduce an entire human being generally evokes condemnation. Using a genetic test to determine whether a person is at increased risk for colon cancer seems prudent because early colonoscopy can target a malignancy for removal before it becomes lethal, but genetic testing for incurable diseases such as Huntington or Alzheimer disease may have psychosocial consequences that outweigh any potential benefit. Antiageing technologies have a tremendous marketing appeal, but there are significant limitations to their benefits and lack of regulatory control on their use. (p. xi)

And what followed from the Preface were the contrasting perspectives by a commendable list of scholars, some extolling the positive elements of extended longevity and the potential for greater quality of life, others examining such ethical quandaries as presymptomatic genetic testing, therapeutic cloning, anti-ageing technologies, and the transhumanist (and posthumanist) movement. Many of these issues will be examined in more detail as we encounter the transition of post ageing into the radical version of the curvature and review the exemplars for [5.5] and beyond. But we think the most important issue that emerges from this publication relates to the theme of "ensuring the equitable distribution of life-extending products and services in a diverse ageing society" (Read et al. 2008; p. xiii). We also think that this represents the greatest challenge and barrier to a full societal understanding and acceptance of the emergent radical version as a part of the nascent view in the study of ageing. Once these issues are addressed in a comprehensive manner (both ethically and equitably), then we foresee the curvature moving beyond [5.4] and into the radical version of [5.5 and >] of the inflection point (and beyond). Thus, we are in agreement with Sprott's (2008) assessment in his chapter titled, "Reality Check: What is Genetic Research on Ageing Likely to Produce, and What are the Ethical and Clinical Implications of Those Advances?", in which he succinctly states the issue and the challenge,

> This question of resource allocation is *the* central ethical question we face in this discussion.At bottom, the issue is not age. Age is just one of the markers we use to discriminate when we allocate resources of any type, including the benefits of scientific advances and expensive medical treatments. Ultimately, the question is how we will allocate the great opportunities we will see as a result of a better understanding of our biology, not whether we can stop that progress. (p. 8)

Aside from the critical issue of "resource allocation," the other ethical conundrums in the "post ageing" inflection point are related to both the experience of the ageing process as a *natural and inevitable outcome* of human development (should it be?) and to the *prospect of mortality* as a part of the human condition (should it be?).

These two dimensions of the post ageing inflection point are hugely controversial and highly provocative and thus reflect the emotionally charged, ethically challenged, and technologically possible landscape of the radical version [5.5 and >] of this positive curvature. The last chapter in the book by Rosemarie Tong (2008), "A Lonely New World—Or Me, Myself, and I," sets the tone for the purported need to establish some boundaries in how fast and how far we (as a society) and those in the health care professions should (or are willing to) go in developing biotechnological therapies. Tong (2008) hoped to establish and elucidate both the nuances of science and the moral practice of medicine in this regard. Is biotechnology supposed to make people happy—or healthy? And supposedly there is a chasm between the two motivations for conducting science and engageing in the development of technological advancements. Tong (2008) placed the same structure of that moral compass against the backdrop of the ageing process—not so much in regards to happiness or health, but mortality or immortality.

Tong (like Read et al. 2008) was seeking a boundary, some sort of firewall, a demarcation of what is needed versus wanted (see Joyce and Loe 2009), what is possible versus pragmatic, what is assistive and what is enhanced, or even overcome, in the domain of biotechnology; yet the same concerns and issues are at stake with the entire landscape of the advancing technologies similar to what Garreau (2005) proposed his "Heaven," "Hell," and "Prevail" scenarios associated with the GRIN categories. The "Prevail" scenario represents the "middle ground" of the debate and activity where humans will seek some limits and guidelines to what is, based on "good" principles and ethical bearings instead of being misguided or dangerous to human welfare. The issues of ethics, morality, limits, purpose, meaning, significance, and the process of science bring us to the crossroads where the *moderate* version [5.1 to 5.4] of the inflection point will cross over to the *radical* version [5.5 and >] of the curvature and towards the activities and literature that will propel the movement onward to Post Ageing (ageing as an *artifact*). But the crossing over is not a simple bridge or even necessarily a smooth transition. Furthermore, we do not want to leave the reader with the impression that there is necessarily a demarcation between the moderate and radical versions of the curvature; rather, the incremental points ([5.1], [5.2], [5.3], [5.4] and so on) noted in the literature represent significant precursors or "portals" toward the radical version and not just a separate category of technology and ageing issues.

The transition toward the radical version [5.5 and >] has energized the dialogue about the goals and values of science and technology. For example, in the year 2002, there were two publications heralding the onset of the varied perspectives, even polemics, associated with the developments of biotechnology. On one hand, Fukuyama (2002) pondered the negative consequences that may emerge from the biotechnology revolution, especially as they relate to the political structures associated with liberal democracy. On the other hand, there were the proclamations of Stock (2002) who argued that the biotechnology revolution is inevitable and that by the end of this millennium, "we would change ourselves enough to become much more than simply human" (p. 5). Stock (2002) further argued that extended life spans (based on a germ line procedure) would benefit both the individual and society,

> Longer and more vital life spans would not only have personal consequences, they would also enrich society. The family cycle of pain and disruption from old age and death is clear to everyone, but economists try to be more specific. William Nordhaus, an economist at Yale University, estimates that half the increase in the standard of living in the United States during the past century is due to the rise in longevity that has lengthened our active lives. The benefits to society of extending our vital years are as a clear as the burdens of prolongeing our decrepitude. We require decades of education and experience to learn to handle ourselves effectively in the world, but we tire and fade all too quickly. Added years of health would lessen the drain. If youth is wasted on the young, then why not see what the old can do with it? (p. 95–96)

Despite the fact that technology and ageing have become irrevocably interconnected (see Joyce and Loe 2009), the threads from previous prevailing views ([1.0], [2.0], [3.0], [4.0]) are still present and guiding our interpretations of the emergent inflection point of post ageing [5.0]. Thus, as the radical version of the inflection point gains momentum, we are increasingly seeing the evidence of the shock waves and turbulence from where science and metaphysics collide (see Tauber 2009): in scholarly journals (e.g., *Journal of Medicine and Philosophy*, *Rejuvenation Research*), in popular fiction (see Bakker 2009; Houellebecq 2005; Shteyngart 2010), in books (here listed by publication date, *The Shattered Self: The End of Natural Selection,* Baldi 2001; *Wondergenes: Genetic Enhancement and the Future of Society*, Mehlman 2003; *Beyond Therapy: Biotechnology and the Pursuit of Happiness*, Kass 2004; *Is Human Nature Obsolete? Genetics, Bioengineering, and the Future of the Human Condition*, Baillie & Casey, 2005; *Genesis Redux: Essays in the History and Philosophy of Artificial Life*, Riskin 2007; *Enhancing Evolution: The Ethical Case for Making Better People*, Harris 2007; *The Case Against Perfection: Ethics in the Age of Genetic Engineering*, Sandel 2007; *Just Genes: The Ethics of Genetics Technologies*, Barash 2008; *The Price of Perfection: Individualism and Society in the Era of Biomedical Enhancement*, Mehlman 2009; *Human Enhancement*, Savulescu, and Bostrom 2009; *Can We Live Forever? A Sociological and Moral Inquiry*, Turner 2009; *Eternity Soup: Inside the Quest to End Ageing*, Critser 2010; *The Youth Pill: Scientists at the Brink of an Anti-Ageing Revolution,* Stipp 2010; *Long for This World: The Strange Science of Immortality*, Weiner, 2010; *Selling the Fountain of Youth: How the Anti-Ageing Industry Made a Disease Out of Getting Old –and Made Billions*, Weintraub 2010), in film (see *Blade Runner, EternalSunshine of the Spotless Mind, Gattaca, Matrix trilogy, Twelve Monkeys, Total Recall, Terminator series, Minority Report,To Age or Not to Age*, (a documentary), trade magazines, and on the internet via a plethora of web sites and blogs (e.g., *Institute for Emergeing Ethics & Technologies, IEET*).

In the study of the ageing process, we are convinced that there will be the need for more panel groups, conferences, special issues of journal publications, and edited books to address the science, morality, and ethics of the intersection of ageing and technology in a balanced and interdisciplinary fashion (see Farrant

2009; Joyce and Loe 2009; Partridge et al. 2009; Temkin 2009). This discourse, consensus, and intervention need to occur now as the radical version [5.5 and >] already has significant momentum worldwide. The entire enterprise of biotechnology, artificial intelligence, robotics, and nanotechnology (as well as nanomedicine) is a sleeping giant that has awakened, and the speed of its delivery and implementation in both research and development laboratories—and then in individual and societal application—is staggering and overwhelming (see Joyce and Loe 2009).

But our call for dialogical intervention and policy guidelines now does not mean that there has been a vacuum of literature on the subject matter, rather the call is targeted to those in the field of gerontology and those who identify themselves as scholars and investigators in the field of ageing to appreciate and understand both the momentum and the implications of the inflection point of "post ageing" intimately connected to both the *moderate* and *radical* versions. Although not every previous publication associated with the radical version has necessarily addressed "ageing issues" per se, it is hoped that this will indicate the need for gerontologists to stay abreast of the burgeoning literature on the GRIN technologies. It is also proposed that every gerontology program in higher education begin to integrate these issues into their existing gerontology courses or offer a special topics course relating to technology and ageing issues. We think every gerontologist should know the differences in values, attitudes, and perspectives among bioconservatives (left and right wing), transhumanists, and technoprogressives, as much as one might expect a gerontologist to know the difference between Medicare, Medicaid, and Medigap. Yes, it is a bold request, but just as we are expected to know the nuances of skilled nursing facilities versus assisted living facilities, or the difference between cross-sectional and longitudinal studies, we should also expect to know of the issues surrounding artificial intelligence, nanotechnologies, immortality, robotics, science fiction, cybernetics, futurology, post-biological, singularity, methuselarity, transhumanism, and posthumanism (de Grey and Rae 2007; DeLashmutt 2006; Derkx 2009).

References

Bakker, R. S. (2009). *Neuropath*. New York: Tom Doherty Associates Book.

Baldi, P. (2001). *The shattered self: the end of natural evolution*. Cambridge, MA: The MIT Press.

Barash, C. I. (2008). *Just genes: The ethics of genetic technologies*. Westport, CT: Praeger.

Burdick, D. C. & Kwon, S. (Eds.).*Gerontechnology: Growing old in a technological society*. Springfield, IL: Charles C. Thomas Publishers.

Critser, G. (2010). *Eternity soup: inside the quest to end ageing*. New York: Harmony Books.

de Grey, A. D. N. J., & Rae, M. (2007). *Ending ageing: the rejuvenation breakthrough that could reverse human ageing in our lifetime*. New York: St. Martin's Press.

DeLashmutt, M. W. (2006). A better life through information technology? The techno-theological eschatology of posthuman speculative science (Perspectives on techno-science and human nature). *Zygon, 41*, 267–287.

Derkx, P. (2009). Engineering substantially prolonged human life spans: Biotechnological enhancement and ethics. In R. Edmondson & H. Kondratowitz (Eds.), *Valuing older people: A humanist approach to ageing* (pp. 177–198). Bristol, UK: The Policy Press.

Farrant, A. (2009). The fair innings argument and increasing life spans. *Journal of Medical Ethics, 35*, 53–56.

Fukuyama, F. (2002). *Our posthuman future: consequences of the biotechnology revolution*. New York: Farrar, Straus and Giroux.

Garreau, J. (2005). *Radical evolution: The promise and peril of enhancing our minds, our bodies—and what it means to be human*. New York: Broadway Random House.

Harris, J. (2007). *Enhancing evolution: The ethical case for making better people*. Princeton, NJ: Princeton University Press.

Houellebecq, M. (2005). *The possibility of an island*. London: Weidenfeld & Nicolson.

Joyce, K., & Loe, M. (2009). A sociological approach to ageing, technology and health. *Sociology of Health and Illness, 32*(2), 171–180.

Kass, L. (2004). *Beyond therapy: Biotechnology and the pursuit of happiness (a report of the president's council on bioethics)*. New York: Dana Press.

Lesnoff-Caravaglia, G. (2004). Ethical realities: The old, the new, and the virtual. In D. C. Burdick & S. Kwon (Eds.), *Gerontechnology: Growing old in a technological society* (pp. 241–255). Springfield, IL: Charles C. Thomas Publishers.

Lesnoff-Caravaglia, G. (2007a). *Gerontechnology: Growing old in a technological society*. Springfield, IL: Charles C. Thomas Publishers.

Lesnoff-Caravaglia, G. (2007b). Gerontechnology: The challenge. In G. Lesnoff-Caravaglia (Ed.), *Gerontechnology: Growing old in a technological society*. Springfield, IL: Charles C. Thomas Publishers.

Mehlman, M. J. (2003). *Wondergenes: Genetic enhancement and the future of society*. Bloomington, ID: Indiana University Press.

Mehlman, M. J. (2009). *The price of perfection: Individualism and society in the era of biomedical enhancement*. Baltimore, MD: The Johns Hopkins University Press.

Nejat, G., Nies, M., & Sexton, T. R. (2010). An interdisciplinary team for the design and integration of assistive robots in health care applications. *Home Health Care Management and Practice, 22*(2), 104–110.

Partridge, B., Underwood, M., Lucke, J., Bartlett, H., & Hall, W. (2009). Ethical concerns in the community about technologies to extend human life span. *The American Journal of Bioethics, 9*(12), 68–76.

Pollack, M. E. (2005). Intelligent technology for an ageing population: The use of AI to assist elders with cognitive impairment. *AI Magazine, 26*(2), 9–24.

Read, C. Y., Green, R. C., & Smyer, M. A. (Eds.). (2008). *Ageing, biotechnology, and the future*. Baltimore, MD: The Johns Hopkins University Press.

Riskin, J. (Ed.). (2007). *Genesis redux: Essays in the philosophy and philosophy of artificial life*. Chicago: University of Chicago Press.

Sandel, M. J. (2007). *The case against perfection: Ethics in the age of genetic engineering*. Cambridge, MA: Harvard University Press (Belknap Press).

Savulescu, J., & Bostrom, N. (2009). *Human enhancement*. New York: Oxford University Press.

Shteyngart, G. (2010). *Super sad true love story*. New York: Random House.

Sprott, R. L. (2008). Reality check: What is genetic research on ageing likely to produce, and what are the ethical and clinical implications of those advances? In C. Y. Read, R. C. Green, & M. A. Smyer (Eds.), *Ageing, biotechnology, and the future*. Baltimore: The Johns Hopkins University Press.

Stipp, D. (2010). *The youth pill: Scientists at the brink of an anti-ageing revolution*. New York: Current (Penguin).

Stock, G. (2002). *Redesigning humans: Our inevitable genetic future*. Boston: Houghton Mifflin Co.

Tauber, A. I. (2009). *Science and the quest for meaning*. Waco, TX: Baylor University Press.

Temkin, L. S. (2009). Is living longer living better? *Journal of applied philosophy, 25*(3), 193–210.

Tong, R. (2008). A lonely new world—Or me, myself, and I. In C. Y. Read, R. C. Green, & M. A. Smyer (Eds.), *Ageing, biotechnology, and the future*. Baltimore: Johns Hopkins Press.

Turner, B. S. (2009). *Can we live forever? A sociological and moral inquiry*. New York: Anthem Press.

Weiner, J. (2010). *Long for this world: The strange science of immortality*. New York: HarperCollins.

Weintraub, A. (2010). *Selling the fountain of youth: How the anti-ageing industry made a disease out of getting old-and made billions*. New York: Basic Books.

Chapter 6
[5.5 and >] Radical Versions of the Inflection Point and Positive Derivative

Abstract The idea of ageing will have become associated with an experience that was in the past, and humans will have moved beyond the process of ageing into a vastly different living experience permeated by qualitative enhancements and bioengineering. With post ageing, there is the expectation of a longevity that would surpass what we now associate with the "maximum life span" of our species.

Keywords Ageing · Debate · Ageing exemplar · Biodemography of ageing · Bioengineering · Biogerontology · Biological determinants of ageing · Biomedicine · Extended life span · GRIN technologies · Human existence · Life extension · Maximum life span · Prolongevity

6.1 Radical Versions of the Inflection Point

To set the stage for the radical version of the [5.0] inflection point and to indicate the continuation of the positive derivative (and curvature), we will directly state the exemplar for [5.5] and then expound on the historical context for the emergence of this exemplar and others. Then we will examine the philosophical and scientific foundations that surround the exemplar and then foray into one rapid developing angle that captures the emergent (soon to be prevailing) view of post ageing.

The exemplar for [5.5] is *Ending Ageing: The Rejuvenation Breakthroughs That Could Reverse Human Ageing in Our Lifetime* by de Grey and Rae (2007). Before we examine some of the contextual issues leading up to this exemplar, we want to directly state the rationale for selecting this controversial and provocative title as the key representative of the tipping point away from the moderate version and critical momentum toward (and as the portal into) the radical version of the [5.0] inflection point. The primary reason for choosing the book by de Grey and Rae (2007) is that it clearly represents a *mainstreaming* of the radical version of

K.F. Felsted and S.D. Wright, *Toward Post Ageing*,
Healthy Ageing and Longevity 1, DOI 10.1007/978-3-319-09051-1_6

post ageing into the hands of the both the professional and the layman in terms of articulating the role of rejuvenation therapies targeted at the molecular and cellular level of the human organism. While there have been many other publications prior to this one by de Grey which present and advocate "anti-ageing" strategies, none have defined and expressed the nuances of biotechnology as effectively and as provocatively as Aubrey de Grey. The book *Ending Ageing: The Rejuvenation Breakthroughs That Could Reverse Human Ageing in Our Lifetime* (de Grey and Rae 2007) is therefore recognized as the exemplar and the gateway publication that captures the radical version of the inflection point. We also propose that de Grey's benchmark publication builds the interconnections with an array of other dimensions of the GRIN technologies (Garreau 2005), which will be discussed in greater detail in the next several sections. But first, we will present some historical, contextual and philosophical factors that help to set the foundation for the emergence of the [5.5] exemplar and for what is possible in the near future for the GRIN technologies, especially as they relate to the study of ageing.

6.2 From Biogerontology to Post Ageing

Earlier in this book, we presented some historical exemplars regarding the [1.0] inflection point (ageing with *reflection*) as it related to the metaphysical issues and ageing by noting the "long grey line" of deep historical roots that originated in the mythology of the Greek and Roman era (see Wright 2008). The interest in the physiological dimensions of the ageing process has a fascinating history as well, but perhaps not as historically deep as the metaphysical dimension. For example, there was the curious 1921 publication by Dodd (1921), *Old Age: Its Cause and Prevention,* which appears to be a provocative precursor to the Jack LaLanne school for living well into the later years. Dodd, who at the age of fifty claimed to have completely broken down physically but then "reversed" his ageing process through a regimen of exercise and diet matched the fabled miracle of Faust by changing an old body into a new one. There was also Hall's (1922) *Senescence: The Last Half of Life* and another book, titled *Old Age: The Major Involution: The Physiology and Pathology of the Ageing Process*, by Warthin (1930). Warthin proclaimed that the involution associated with the later years was a "tragicomedy" which would only create a greater number of individuals who would reach their eighties and nineties, "more or less useless" since they enter into a second childhood.

Moving forward, we could also seek guidance in *Ageing, the Biology of Senescence* by Comfort (1964) and we certainly have to acknowledge the benchmark publication for biogerontology, Hayflick's (1994) *How and Why We Age*. Hayflick's book is considered a classic mainstream publication for biogerontology. It also included a foreword by Robert Butler suggesting that many ethical dilemmas would have to be addressed before engaging in lofty scientific goals and tampering with the clocks that govern ageing. But that was then—and this is now, and the game (and the literature) has changed dramatically since 1994, such that there appears to be much more interest in *How Not to Age and Why Not* (meaning, Do we have to age at all?). Hayflick has come from being one of the few voices addressing the issues of biogerontology (with his 1994 publication) to being one of its leading spokespersons (see Hayflick's 2009 leadership with symposium presentation "Ageing Is No Longer an Unsolved Biological Problem" at the World Congress of Gerontology and Geriatrics in Paris, France), but he is also actively engaged in the defensive posture of defining *biogerontology* against anti-ageing medicine, or prolongevity, or the disease model orientation of many scientists, or the burgeoning activity (both scientific and market-based) that seeks to extend the human life span. For example, in an interview with the publication *Technology Review*, Leonard Hayflick made it very clear that understanding the *cause* of ageing does not necessarily mean that there is a "cure" to the ageing process,

> TR: So it doesn't imply that there is a solution to ageing?
> LH: Why would you want to do that?
> TR: Some people would like to slow or halt the ageing process.
> LH: They haven't thought about the consequences. We relate to each other by perceptions of differences in age, which would be destroyed if some chose to increase their longevity and some did not. The social, political, and economic discontinuities that would occur would be enormous. People who say they want extended longevity say they want it to be so when life satisfaction is greatest. Yet they won't know [when that is] until late in life. If you're in your eighties and you decide you want life extended when you were happier, at fifty, it's no longer possible. (*Technology Review*, 7/1/2009; see article at http://www.technologyreview.com/biomedicine/22954.)

In essence, Hayflick (1994, 2004) was perfectly comfortable in drawing a line knowing the underlying issues with ageing (the how and the why) and embracing the natural order and limits that are essentially built into the human organism (i.e., "the Hayflick Limit") rather than entertaining any efforts that are "highly improbable" in terms of extending life beyond the biologically determined life span. Furthermore, Hayflick was very specific about where the focus of research and large funding opportunities should go in ageing during his interview,

> TR: Why is it so important to distinguish between ageing and the diseases of ageing?
> LH: You cannot learn about the fundamental biology of ageing by studying disease processes. Resolving age-associated diseases tells us nothing about the fundamental biology of ageing, just as the resolution of childhood diseases, such as polio and childhood anemia, did not tell us one iota about childhood development.
> (Retrieved from http://www.technologyreview.com/biomedicine/22954/page2/.)

And yet, this perspective of Hayflick drew a response from Ray Kurzweil (who will be covered more in this section) about a week later in the same publication (*Technology Review* via their blog site) who replied with a rebuttal titled, "How to

Combat Ageing" (July 2009). Kurzweil's (2009) viewpoint runs counter to Hayflick's perspectives in that Kurzweil is a complete and unabashed devotee of the promise of bioengineering potential and believes that Hayflick's "science" focuses on "limits" ("the Hayflick limit") and that he is hampered and hamstrung by a conventional linear thinking that expects, "...that the slow pace of the past will characterize the future." And so Kurzweil (2009) argued that,

> ...the reality of progress in information technology is exponential, not linear...We do not yet have all of the knowledge and tools to do this with the human body, but that knowledge is growing exponentially.

We think the best way to frame the debate between Hayflick and Kurzweil is to review once again our heuristic of inflection points as a tool to understand how scholars can operate within vastly differing viewpoints while sharing an interest in biogerontology. As you recall, the proposed inflection points were designated as,

[1.0]: Philosophy of Ageing (ageing as a *reflection*)
[2.0]: Bio-medical diseases of ageing (ageing as a *problem*)
[3.0]: Demographics of Ageing (ageing as a *challenge*)
[4.0]: Optimal Ageing (ageing as a *reward*)
[5.0]: Post Ageing (ageing as an *artifact*)

and Hayflick's scholarship record is very much connected to inflection point [2.0] and [4.0] with his emphasis on biological determinants of ageing (although it should be noted that Hayflick has clearly stated the need to separate the biological process of ageing from disease processes) and that ageing is a "problem" that can be overcome by focusing scientific research on the underlying process of ageing—and not exclusively on disease per se. Hayflick would like to see advances in science lead to a better quality of life so humans can live out the natural order of life until (but not past) the point of maximum life span. In other words, life expectancy should be optimized ([4.0]) up until the point of the natural "limit" endowed within *Homo sapiens* such that anything that would focus beyond that "limit" is simply not scientifically feasible, nor would it be desirable for our species. And this is a critical demarcation point—the inflection point that Hayflick operates within. Alternately, Kurzweil (2009) clearly operates in the [5.0] inflection point and curvature that has a different prevailing viewpoint about so-called "limits" and the inevitability of the ageing process and maximum life span. Most importantly, the prevailing viewpoint associated with [5.x], especially with [5.4] and greater (the radical versions) carries forward the scholarship and application to lead us toward the full realization of post ageing. Kurzweil (like Aubrey de Grey and many others) is deeply embedded in the promotion and use of radical versions of the GRIN technologies (Garreau 2005) which also serve as the mechanism to realize the time in the future in which ageing will be an seen as artifact. In other words, the idea of ageing will have become associated with an *experience* that was in the past, and humans will have moved beyond the process of ageing into a vastly different living experience permeated by qualitative enhancements and bioengineering. With post ageing, there is the expectation of a longevity that would surpass what we now associate with the "maximum life span" of our species. Here is Kurzweil (2009) indicating (from the blog posting in *Technology Review* (http://www.technologyreview.com/blog/guest/23802/) the promise of technology as it relates to interventions in sustaining the quality of life.

> The most important perspective in my view is that health, medicine, and biology is now an information technology, whereas it used to be hit or miss. We not only have the (outdated) software that biology runs on (our genome), but we have the means of changing that software (our genes) in a mature individual with such technologies as RNA interference and new forms of gene therapy that do not trigger the immune system…We can design interventions on computers and test them out on increasingly sophisticated biological simulators. One of my primary themes is that information technology grows exponentially, in sharp contrast to the linear growth of hit or miss approaches that have characterized medicine up until recently. As such, these technologies will be a million times more powerful in 20 years (by doubling in power and price performance each year). The genome project, incidentally, followed exactly this trajectory.

Kurzweil's perspective is further elaborated in his book, co-authored by Kurzweil and Grossman (2009) *Transcend: Nine Steps to Living Well Forever* in which the authors "promise to reverse ageing, extend your life span, and maintain vitality forever." The working premise of the book, as well as Kurzweil's strategy for the near future, is that if people follow the guidelines ("the nine steps") then they will remain healthy enough, and live long enough, to then "take full advantage of the biotech and nanotech miracles of tomorrow." Kurzweil and Grossman (2009) has gone on record to state that he believes that "immortality" is only 20 years away according to his theory, "The Law of Accelerating Returns". This "law" presumes that our understanding of genes and computer technology is increasing; thus, nanotechnologies will be able to replace vital organs in human body systems.

Needless to say, not everyone is in agreement with such prognostications about the future and the promise of reversing ageing—the complete realization of post ageing—for both scientific and ethical reasons. Thus, before we move forward into the radical versions [5.5 and >] of the inflection point of *Post Ageing*, (e.g., *Ending Ageing: The Rejuvenation Breakthroughs That Could Reverse Human Ageing in Our Lifetime* (de Grey and Rae 2007), it is necessary to briefly review the literature that has critically examined the merits of anti-ageing medicine, life extension, and the quest for immortality. This will help to provide an important counterweight to the burgeoning line of literature that is promoting a more *optimistic* perspective at the intersection of biotechnology and ageing. This may serve as the keystone feature for the prevailing view of inflection point [5.x] versus that of the [4.0] inflection point: the supposed benefits of GRIN technologies do not only optimize ageing [4.0] and fulfill a complete life span existence ("natural order of human life to maximum life span"), but actually surpass and exceed the maximum life span for Homo sapiens. This leads to the possibility that human existence may be transcended by some other entity with far greater intelligence and survival potential than what exists for the organic "limits" of the human body. This is what makes the [5.x] inflection point and the curvature representing [5.5 and >] so vastly different in its prevailing view than that of [4.0]: optimal ageing. It is important to state that not all scholars who are in support of using the

GRIN technologies are in agreement about the so-called "optimistic" end result for either humans or the planet from an economic and ecological perspective (see Garreau 2005 with the *Heaven, Hell,* and *Prevail* scenarios). Therefore, the following material will help address some of the historical, philosophical and technological dimensions of the [5.x] curvature as it relates the activities from biogerontology to post ageing.

6.3 Historical, Philosophical, and Technological Dimensions of Post Ageing

While there are numerous places to begin this part of the discussion, we choose to start with an essay by Jay Olshansky (1998) in the journal *Population and Development Review* titled, "On the Biodemography of Ageing: A Review Essay", which is actually a review of the edited book by Wachter and Finch (1997), titled *Between Zeus and the Salmon: The Biodemography of Longevity*. We believe the essay by Olshansky (1998) is a comprehensive start point for the essential questions that surround biogerontology:

(1) Why do we age? (Or, why are we not immortal?)
(2) How do we age? (Or, what are biological mechanisms that lead human development into senescence and ultimately death?)
(3) When do we age? (Or, why do ageing and death occur when they do in various species and why is there variation in ages at death between and within species?)

Olshansky (1998) then set the stage for further debate (as well as tension among various camps within biogerontology) by positing an interesting philosophical perspective on the role of mortality in humans, the prospect of life extension, and the direction of any future research. Here Olshansky (1998) provided critique to the "overemphasis" found in the biologically oriented chapters that explained decelerating mortality at older ages among humans and the rise of in the number of centenarians among humans in modern times,

> To be sure, both are interesting phenomena. However, they are largely irrelevant in genetically heterogeneous populations like humans where the majority of any birth cohort contains neither the genotype nor the practical means to survive as long as the population's longevity outliers. At this point the interest in centenarians should be at the level of identifying alleles that favor extreme longevity, as Finch suggests in his chapter. An understanding of post reproductive survival in humans requires a focus on the vast majority who die between the ages of 60 and 100 and on the alleles that influence their deaths rather than on the small segment of every birth cohort with the potential to survive old age. (p. 390)

From this point, we move forward with reports from the Government Accountability Office (e.g., 'Health Products for Seniors: "Anti-Ageing" Products Pose Potential for Physical and Economic Harm,' GAO-01-1129) regarding the dubious claims of many products promoted as "anti-ageing" or "cure-all" claims. (Government Accountability Office [GAO] 2001). These are typically targeted to senior citizens and may actually cause physical or economic harm. This seemed to be the sentinel report that invited more scholars to jump in on the topic, for example, an article by Olshansky et al. (2002a) in the publication *Scientific American* titled, "No Truth to the Fountain of Youth", as well as another article by Olshansky et al. (2002b) in the *Journal of Gerontology: Biological Sciences* titled, "Position statement on human ageing" . This last article was endorsed by 51 leading gerontologists (both articles followed closely on the heels of the book authored by Olshansky and Carnes (2001) *The Quest for Immortality: Science at the Frontiers of Ageing*). A special issue of *Generations* (Winter 2001–2002) published many good articles on the topic: "Anti-Ageing: Are You For It Or Against It?", and Binstock (2003) in his article in *The Gerontologist*, "The War on 'Anti-ageing Medicine'", according to Vincent (2003) in a review essay in the journal *Ageing & Society* titled "What's at Stake in the 'War on Anti-ageing Medicine'?" "contextualizes the anti-ageing debate in the scientific and research-funding politics that underlies American gerontology's growth". Vincent further proposed that Binstock suggested that "the gerontological establishment is engaged in 'boundary work' to discredit rivals in the anti-ageing medicine movement" (p. 678), and, in particular, to deny the scientific legitimacy of the *American Academy of Anti-Ageing Medicine* (A4M) (Vincent 2003; and see Binstock 2004). The year 2003 is then topped off with the book, *Merchants of Immortality: Chasing the Dream of Human Life Extension* by Hall (2003) who examined the intersection of biology and business as it related to regenerative medicine and human life extension (see also Atala et al. 2010). Hall's (2003) account is balanced but the overall assessment from his point of view is the *inevitability* of biotechnologies as a major force in the 21st century,

> ...even without dramatic life extension medicines, even without "practical immortality," this is where we are headed already. The genomics revolution, personalized medicine, stem cell therapy, and other advances in regenerative medicine—the technologies may take decades to ripen, but they are already in train. (p. 352)

So as you can see by the few examples in the literature thus far (from Olshansky's 1998 publication through the year 2003), the so-called "war" had begun and the choosing of sides in the debate was underway in terms of where one would stand on the issue of "anti-ageing medicine" and the ethics of human life extension. The following year, the debate and discussion (e.g., see Stock and Callahan 2004) continued with a Special Section of the *Journal of Gerontology: Biological Sciences* entitled "Anti-Ageing Medicine" with Jay Olshansky et al. (2004) serving as guest editors. They reiterated their stance in the introduction that,

> In spite of numerous claims to the contrary, there is no empirical evidence to support the claim that humans can be modified by any means, nor is there evidence that it is possible to measure biological age, or that anti-ageing products extend the duration of life. (p. 513)

And yet Olshansky et al. (2004) believed that the onslaught of media attention (primarily in print, radio, and television; strangely, they made no mention of the Internet) on the topic of anti-ageing medicine warranted further manuscripts to separate the hype from the reality. This special issue (Vol.59A, No.6) addressed three topics: (1) *Anti-Ageing Medicine: The History*; (2) *Debates* (on whether or not ageing is a disease and the societal implications of modifying the biological rate of ageing; and (3) *Ageing: The Reality* (where various researchers discussed in general what was currently known about ageing, its measurement, and the extreme tail of the human survival distribution). We found the three most intriguing articles in the special issue to be written by Haber (2004), Binstock (2004), and Post (2004), all elaborating on relevant issues connected to the [5.x] inflection point of post ageing. For example, Haber (2004) offers a fascinating historical accounting of "the continual search for the fountain youth" but also submits a scathing indictment of the current anti-age movement, which appears to repeat the campaigns of the past,

> From the perspective of history, then, the new fountain of youth may not simply be offering its supplicants the hope of fewer wrinkles and a more active sex life. In both its formula for continued youth and its contempt for elderly people, the anti-age movement, like its late 19th century and early 20th century counterparts, tends to demean and marginalize the very process of growing old. (p. 521)

Haber (2004) seems to be convinced that the more recent activities promoting "anti-ageing medicines" are akin to subtle, or not so subtle, ageism, and although we see her point and think it is a worthy message for all of us in the field of gerontology to consider, we are not convinced the advancement of GRIN technologies (as opposed to "anti-ageing medicines") is necessarily driven or motivated by the desire to "demean and marginalize the very process of growing old."On the other hand, many of the GRIN technologies do appear to be interested in modulating the process of ageing and the consequences thereof, but we would like to submit as a counter-message to Haber (2004) that these technologies also have the capacity to ameliorate the physical and cognitive impairments and suffering associated with later life. It is important to carefully scrutinize, and differentiate between, the interventions that purport to be "anti-ageing medicines" versus the varied technologies that will possibly alleviate suffering and enhance life—making it both longer and better.

Binstock's (2004) article in the special issue, "Anti-Ageing Medicine and Research: A Realm of Conflict and Profound Societal Implications" is quite simply a brilliant piece of scholarship. We agree with his assessment that there is a need for "public discussion" on the varied dimensions of biogerontology, anti-ageing medicine, and the topic of "prolongevity", since much of the theory and research, and thus the vocabulary and currency by which activities are communicated, have common ground despite the heated debates. At minimum, there is a need to differentiate among the labels and goals of the various camps and determine what science is being conducted (versus pseudo-science); there is also a need to examine the social consequences of attainment of prolongevity interventions. In that regard, Binstock (2004) advances "Three Prolongevity Paradigms" to organize and categorize the various dimensions (see also Carnes and Olshansky 2007). While we wish that Binstock would have avoided using the term "paradigm" (as it simply adds more confusion to the already overused, even misused, word in our field) the purpose and design of his analysis (The Three Paradigms) is extremely relevant to the use of the heuristic of *inflection points* and to the [5.x] curvature of post ageing. Binstock's (2004) three "prolongevity" paradigms are:

(1) Compression of Morbidity
(2) Decelerated Ageing
(3) Arrested Ageing

The first paradigm (and Binstock refers to this one as the most "conservative") addresses the activities associated with a *compression of morbidity* which can increase life expectancy such that humans can "live long lives free of chronic disease and disability, and then die rather quickly as we reach the limits of the human species life span because we are "worn out" from the fundamental processes of ageing" (p. 530). It is important to note that within this "paradigm" the focus is on increasing life *expectancy*, but because the paradigm assumes a fixed genetic fixed life *span*, the period of infirmity is shortened, there is no research activity that attempts to lengthen the maximum life *span*. In the context of the heuristic of inflection points, this "paradigm" reflects the inflection point of [2.0] Bio-medical diseases of Ageing (ageing as a *problem*), which captures the focused procedures of the bio-medical model.

The second "paradigm", *decelerated ageing*, captures the research interventions in which the ageing processes are slowed and average life expectancy and/or maximum life span are increased. Here the goal is to maximize the optimal conditions for ageing well and delay the onset of later-life frailty (which is still inevitable, but occurring at a later age than previously). In our opinion (and in the context of the heuristic of inflection points), this "paradigm" falls under and reflects the inflection point of [4.0] Optimal Ageing (ageing as a *reward*). It is interesting to note that Binstock refers to the work of Aubrey de Grey in relation to the second paradigm but it is the third "paradigm", *arrested ageing*, where the work of de Grey is prominently highlighted.

The main attribute of *arrested ageing* is that the processes of ageing are *reversed* in adults—and the goal is to "restore vitality and function to those who have lost them, akin to the rejuvenation theme that has been present in prolongevity myths and quests for millennia" (p. 530). Binstock (2004) acknowledges the work of de Grey as moving toward "negligible senescence" but there is not much discussion on *how* this would be achieved. In other words, Binstock (2004) does not elaborate on the strategies to engineer the "indefinite postponement of ageing." In any case, this "paradigm" falls under the inflection point of [5.0] Post Ageing (ageing as an *artifact*) where strategies are proactively used to reverse the ageing process and increase the human life span beyond the genetic fixed limit, such that "life expectancies of around 1000 years would be attained" (p. 530). This is *not* the first reference to de Grey's work in gerontological journals per se, but in our analysis, the referencing by Binstock (2004) represents a major milestone in indicating de Grey's emergent work as creating a new "paradigm."However, we have previously stated that de Grey and Rae's (2007) later work, *Ending Ageing: The Rejuvenation Breakthroughs That Could Reverse Human Ageing in our Lifetime,* is the benchmark publication for the point of the curvature for the *radical version* [5.5] of the inflection point *Post Ageing.*

The article in the special issue of the *Journal of Gerontology: Biological Sciences (*Vol.59A, No.6) by Post (2004), "Establishing an Appropriate Ethical Framework: The Moral Conversation Around the Goal of Prolongevity", is highly recommended as a primer of the various ethical and philosophical stances (e.g., natural law, equalitarian justice, and beneficence) that intersect with the promise of the deceleration of human ageing. Post (2004) presents an accessible overview of such terms as *posthumanism* (e.g., the view that today's humans will be superseded by superior models) and its equivalent, *transhumanism,* and how these philosophical perspectives embrace both decelerated and reversible ageing (but only as a small part of reengineering human nature). Post (2004) presents an impressive comparison analysis among the ethical viewpoints and offers an interesting conclusion when taking into account the many arguments (see Fukuyama 2002) against biotechnological developments and the prolongevity stance,

> Should we move forward in the 21st century as bold new "cocreators" of our somewhat malleable human nature, or should we accept a more humble approach that endorses a caring and just stewardship over human nature more or less at it is, seeking therapies instead of transformations. At least in decelerated ageing, where therapy and enhancement merge, *science should go forward* in exploring the potential to eradicate the overwhelming morbidity associated with old age. The intended and direct moral goal must be to free older adults from senility and decrepitude, while an indirect side effect would be the addition of good years in which long-lived individual hopefully contribute to the common good through prosocial and generative behaviors that themselves seem to contribute to health and longevity. (p. 539; emphasis added).

Although Post (2004) believes there is reason for caution in embracing biotechnological developments, the conclusion is clear: science should move forward with technologies that would decelerate the ageing process. Goldman et al. (2013), who include Olshansky, in their article entitled "Substantial Health and Economic Returns from Delayed Ageing May Warrant a New Focus for Medical Research," state that "greater investment in research to delay ageing appears to be a highly efficient way to forestall disease, extend healthy life, and improve public health". Again, science should move forward. This, of course, is not the end of the debate on prolongevity—scientifically, ethically or philosophically. For example, there have been numerous publications since the special issue of the *Journal of Gerontology: Biological Sciences* entitled "Anti-Ageing Medicine" (Olshansky et al. 2004) that have continued the discussion (see Baudisch 2008; Carnes and Olshansky 2007; Goldsmith 2008; Hadley et al. 2005; Joyce and Loe 2009; Kampf and Botelho 2009; Martin 2006; Mitteldorf and Pepper 2009; Robine et al. 2006; Rose 2005; Vina et al. 2007). It is especially important to highlight the special edition of *Journal of Ageing Studies,* "The Anti-Ageing

Enterprise: Science, Knowledge, Expertise, Rhetoric and Values," with the guest editors, Vincent et al. (2008) and the special issue of *Journal of Gerontology: Biological Sciences* (Vol. 64A, 2) with articles related to the "Biology of Ageing Summit" and *Medicine Studies*, "Anti-Ageing and Biomedicine: Critical Studies on the Pursuit of Maintaining, Revitalizing and Enhancing Ageing Bodies" with the guest editors, Kampf and Botelho (2009). Given this review of some of the historical, philosophical and technological dimensions surrounding the emergence of the [5.x] curvature as it relates the activities from biogerontology to post ageing, we can now summarize the field at several different levels by using the heuristic of the inflection points through an outline of the key features characterizing perspectives with regards to human life extension, prolongevity, and biogerontology. After this summary outline we will move into the domain of the radical versions [5.5 >] of the inflection point of "postageing," and view the proposed benchmark of *Ending Ageing: The Rejuvenation Breakthroughs That Could Reverse Human Ageing in Our Lifetime* (de Grey and Rae 2007).

6.4 The Use of Inflection Points to Understand the Emergence of Post Ageing

6.4.1 [1.0] Philosophy of Ageing (Ageing as a Reflection)

The classical tradition of the deep reflection on the life course and the ageing process in spiritual, ethical, and philosophical perspectives (e.g., natural law, equalitarianism) is reengaged when centered around the goal of human life extension and prolongevity (DeLashmutt 2006; Mykytyn 2008; Post 2004). "Natural law thinkers [e.g., Leon R. Kass—"Beyond Therapy" and Council on Bioethics] exhort us to live more or less according to nature, and warn that our efforts to depart from what we are will result in new evils that are more perilous than old ones." There should be the acceptance of ageing rather than on its scientific modification (see Joyce and Loe 2009). These perspectives are reminiscent of the Stoic tradition of Seneca's *De Brevitate Vitae* "On the Shortness of Life"; Cicero's *De Senectute*, and Marcus Aurelius's *Meditations.* Thus any attempts at pursuing prolongevity activities in research and application (i.e., reengineering human nature and creating biologically and technologically superior human beings—"posthumanism") is deemed to run counter to natural law tenets and that posthumanism (and its predilections for cybernetics, nanotechnology, genetic enhancement, reproductive cloning, life span extensions) threatens to disrupt the "demographic balances between young and old, and exacerbate the gap between the haves and the have-nots" (see Fukuyama 2002). Finally, Vincent (2003, 2006, 2008) has framed post ageing (and anti-ageing medicine) activities as part of the "crisis" in gerontology in relation to its core values and mission. Vincent (2003) believes that the crisis is "not technological, but cultural" as gerontology falls deeper into the grasp of scientism ("the infallibility of science") and assumes that immortality can be achieved via technological competence (see also Vincent 2006). And here is the consequence, from a philosophical perspective:

> The consequence of this set of beliefs is that science, as culture, misdirects the way in which old age is understood, particularly in the presumption that science potentially can cure death. Rather than valuing life in all its diversity, including its final phase, it leads to misguided allocation of resources to solving the problem of death. The focus on biological failure sets up a cultural construction of old age that generates and prolongs its low esteem. An irredeemable cultural logic is created: if death is soluble, old age represents a failure. (p. 682).

This perspective was also addressed in the work of Joyce and Loe (2009) who are concerned about the demarcation that has been structured with one side assuming ageing is a *given*, but yet technology can assist in adaptations (assistive) and thus lead to empowering the older adult to be an active agent in choosing and creating the kinds of technology desired (thus older adults are viewed as "technogenarians") and the other side where ageing is *not a given*—that is to say, ageing is to be transformed from within—from the inside out—via the matrix of anti-ageing medicine interventions. This perspective raises critical issues of whether or not ageing is viewed as a given or not—and whether or not the "intervention" is internal or external to the ageing body.

6.4.2 [2.0] Bio-Medical Diseases of Ageing (Ageing as a Problem)

This inflection point has arrived at several major crossroads in the past 30 years in terms of its primary focus, scientific goals, and critical assessments of the prevailing view within the inflection point. We have seen the intersection of social policy from a critical gerontology perspective and the condition and needs of the elderly population (i.e., "The Ageing Enterprise") (Estes 1993); the struggle between interest groups for the power to shape the future directions of science within gerontology and geriatrics (i.e., "The Alzheimerization of Ageing," Adleman 1995); the challenge of providing better care for older people with multiple chronic conditions (Norris et al. 2008; Reuben 2007); the numerous medical challenges of improving the quality of a longer life (Michel et al. 2008); and whether we think of ageing as a disease or as a natural part of the life course (Mykytyn 2006a, b).

6.4.3 [3.0] Demography of Ageing (Ageing as a Challenge)

These challenges are then placed into the larger context of whether or not the United States can sustain medical care costs with 77 million baby boomers entering into the older age brackets. Hall (2008) was also concerned that any increased longevity realized could be a

> Pyrrhic victory if those additional years are characterized by inexorable morbidity from chronic illness, frailty-associated disability, and increased lowered quality of life (p. 262).

Yet Hall (2008) also observed that disability rates have been steadily declining about 2 % per year in the United States, approximately twice as fast as longevity is increasing. "Morbidity and disability is indeed being compressed into a smaller time frame near the end of life as predicted by Fries in the 'compression of morbidity' hypothesis" (p. 263), which correlates to one of the "paradigms" proposed by Binstock (2004) related to prolongevity. Here the goal is to understand both the genetic and nongenetic factors that extend life expectancy toward the natural limits of the life span. This is represented by research focused on exceptional longevity associated with centenarians and supercentenarians and the influence of familial factors that appear to privilege centenarian offspring who are more likely to age with better cardiovascular health and lower mortality than their peers (Adams et al. 2008; Perls et al. 2007).

6.5 [4.0] Optimal Ageing (Ageing as a *Reward*)

Research applicable to the next inflection point focuses on the modifiable healthy behaviors (smoking abstinence/cessation, weight management, blood pressure control, and regular exercise) that can enhance life span and good health and function during old age (Yates et al. 2008). The goals are very much connected to the investigation of fundamental processes for *both* the study of the ageing process *and* interventions to compress (or eliminate completely) the morbidity in later life so as to *optimize* the health and well-being of the older adult until the inevitable—the end point known the maximum life span.

6.6 The Questionable Desirability of Immortality

The search for the "fountain of youth" is still ongoing (Olshansky and Carnes 2001), and some see this as related to deeper philosophical (metaphysical) perspectives about the value of youth versus ageing. For example, Haber (2004) has stated that, "From the perspective of history, then, the new fountain of youth may not simply be offering its supplicants the hope of fewer wrinkles and a more active sex life. In both its formula for continued youth and its contempt for elderly people, the anti-age movement, like its late 19th century and early 20th century counterparts, tends to demean and marginalize the very process of growing old" (p. 521). Yet others see the search for the "fountain of youth" as an exercise in futility, especially as it is associated with the "pseudoscience of practitioners and entrepreneurs." Thus, there has been a concentrated effort to create boundaries, even battle lines, between the anti-ageing medicine movement and the gerontological establishment in staking out territory in terms of legitimacy in scientific research (see Binstock 2004; Fishman et al. 2008; Zs-Nagy 2009). In any case, Hayflick (2004) is very clear about the matter (given his definition of the ageing process):

> No intervention will slow, stop, or reverse the ageing process in humans and much of the anti-ageing industry strives to conceal cosmetically the nonpathological changes associated with the ageing phenotype...

Furthermore, Hayflick (2004) is adamant about distinguishing between the phenomena of ageing with its associated diseases and the importance of understanding ageing as a stochastic process not programmed by genes. Hayflick sees "ageing" as a fundamental property of all matter, both living and inanimate. Hayflick (2004) believes that "it is not the fear of ageing but the fear of approaching death that motivates the prolongevists" (p. 578). Hayflick also offered his philosophical perspective on the topic, "If our society would learn to value old age to the same extent as we presently value youth, then the drive to slow, stop, or reverse the ageing process would be as unthinkable as intervening in the developmental processes of our youth. What is desirable, and demonstrably attainable at all times in life, is the prevention of or resolution of pathology" (p. 578). But Mykytyn (2006a) has noted that the emergence and proliferation of anti-ageing medicine since the 1990s situates the process of ageing—rather than "age-associated" disease—as a target for biomedical intervention. Bypassing the notion of disease entirely, anti-ageing proponents argue that biological ageing is the problemand that it no longer matters if ageing is natural since it can be the target of therapy (Mykytyn 2006a, b). Mykytyn (2006a) also noted that the applicability of historical trends to future events is a point of contention such that many mainstream gerontologists see most of the gains in human longevity already realized, while anti-ageing proponents envision a geometric increase in biotechnological knowledge that will lead to dramatic increases in longevity and "practical human immortality." Turner (2004), on the other hand, has suggested that there is no persuasive scientific evidence to suggest that humans are on the verge of becoming "posthuman immortals" and that "...we should ensure that we connect our rhetoric and moral deliberation to realistic conceptions of human biology" (p. 221) (see also Aaron and Schwartz 2004). Anton (2013) suggests that the road to immortality is paved by many and varied players with stakes in different industries. Biotech is affected by business, and Anton argues that media and ego have great effect on this pursuit of ending ageing. And researchers like de Grey (2004) believe that the future is now. de Grey has proposed that actual *repair* (not just retardation of accumulation), via his SENS project, of

> age-related molecular and cellular damage (which consists of seven major categories of 'rejuvenation therapy') appears to be technically feasible and, by its nature, is indefinitely extensible to greater life spans without recourse to further conceptual breakthroughs (p. 724).

de Grey (2004) referred to the threshold of the actualizing of benefits of repairas "actuarial escape velocity" (or AEV), which is the dramatic reduction of age-specific mortality risk and then leap-frogging into (hoped for) future benefits derived from geometric gains in bioengineering. Kurzweil (2009) refers to these "leap-frogging" gains in human longevity (and thus potential for immortality) as "bridges" with the second bridge (of three) associated with the biotechnology revolution (see Kurzweil and Grossman 2009; Mykytyn 2006a, b).

6.7 Motley Views of [5.X]: The Futurists, Optimists, and Realists

But at this point in the literature we arrive at the crossroads for perspectives on human life extension, prolongevity, and biogerontology and it appears that the path taken—or direction to follow for any scholar—hinges on the outlook and predictions for the weighted factor of the roles (if any) that the GRIN technologies will play in shifting the post ageing curvature from *moderate* to *radical* versions. In other words, one can still embrace the moderate version of the inflection point, but see little or no gain from any other advancements in the radical versions simply because there is scant evidence from historical and current trends to suggest anything that would resemble a "heaven" (a la Garreau) or an "actuarial escape velocity" (a la de Grey) or "bridges" or a "singularity" in the near future (a la Kurzweil). While some might see only a "hell" scenario with advances in biotechnology, others see a modest and incremental progress in extending and enhancing human life (the "prevail" scenario). Others have a far more progressive and radical outlook and interpretation of what the future has in store for the human life course—to the point of envisioning "immortality." These various perspectives are associated with the classification of major positions proposed by Carnes and Olshansky (2007): *futurists*, those who believe that immortality is within reach; *optimists*, those who believe life expectancy will rise to 100 years or more in this century; and the *realists*, those who believe (like Carnes and Olshansky) that life expectancy is "unlikely to exceed an average of around 85 years *in the absence of radical advances in the control of the ageing process*—and could even decline in developed countries of the world." (emphasis added) (see also Olshansky and Carnes et al. 2009). Therein lies the wild card for the realist perspective; "in the absence of radical advances in the control of the ageing process." This is exactly the critical element—*radical advances in the control of the ageing process* (e.g., GRIN technologies)—that represents the working assumption, the overriding thesis, the crucial intervention, and the essence of the curvature for the radical version of the inflection point of "post ageing." It is here that we have the "break-point", the critical tipping point, for many of the scholars in the field who have an interest in understanding the limits or manipulating the potential for extending human life beyond the supposed "natural" maximum life span. Thus as Hildt (2009) sees it, research into human ageing has two central foci: geriatric medicine working to reduce the incidence and severity of age-related diseases and disabilities by devising adequate therapeutic and preventive strategies, and biogerontology, bringing about a general retardation of the ageing process and thus increasing the average as well as the maximum human lifespan. In other words, there is the optimization of ageing, the compression of morbidity, the reduction of impairments, and the fulfillment of "well-being" across the entire life course and into the supercentenarian years, but this is either seen and believed to be sufficient/reasonable or it is seen as insufficient/unreasonable. That is, humans have at their disposal and use the belief that the ageing process is either inevitable or malleable; it is a natural process of human development or it is a process to be transcended; it is a function of biological destiny and evolutionary strategy or it is landscape for complete intervention, augmentation, enhancement, and metamorphosis. And so within the [5.0] inflection point of post ageing there is also the crossroads at which the *moderate version* is poised to yield to the *radical version* with all of its power and belief of proponents and practitioners who collectively seek to move past the treating of illness and disability in humans (i.e., medicine as *therapeutic*) and instead embrace the notion of "human enhancement" which conceptually transcends a state of mere health to the alternative goal of improving human function "beyond a normal range" (or into "supernormal enhancements") (Brey 2009, p. 169).

A significant dimension of "human enhancement" is the quest for "ending ageing" through the use of GRIN technologies (or, as Brey (2009) has described it, *human enhancement technologies* (HETs)—and that is the focus of the next section of this book where we continue with the lead exemplar for [5.5 and >] *Ending Ageing: The Rejuvenation Breakthroughs That Could Reverse Human Ageing in Our Lifetime* by de Grey and Rae (2007) and expand on the latest developments on the use of technologies that will influence the ageing process—and ultimately lead to the full expression of post ageing.

6.8 [5.5 and >] Radical Versions of the Inflection Point and Positive Derivative

The radical version of the [5.0] inflection point is characteristically provocative, rebellious, confrontational, and relentless in pursuing and pushing for an alternative outlook of the ageing process compared to the traditional, mainstream view that is typically associated with biogerontology (e.g., via Leonard Hayflick's work). As mentioned earlier, one of the key aspects of the radical version is the evolving view that *something can be done* via targeted interventions to retard and—this is the key element of the radical version—*reverse* the ageing process. In other words, it is not enough to know and understand the process of mammalian ageing; the goal is to eliminate not only "age-related diseases" but also "ageing" itself via promising technologies (e.g., GRIN). Therefore, this becomes the basis for our selection of de Grey's book, *Ending Ageing: The Rejuvenation Breakthroughs That Could Reverse Human Ageing in Our Lifetime* as the lead exemplar for the radical version of post ageing.

Ending Ageing: The Rejuvenation Breakthroughs That Could Reverse Human Ageing in Our Lifetime was published in 2007, but the groundwork for de Grey's perspective and activities for "Strategies for Engineered Negligible Senescence" (SENS) goes back to around 2000. For example, he claims that he first used the phrase "engineered negligible senescence" in his 1999 book, *The Mitochondrial Free Radical Theory of Ageing,* and then further elaborated on "ENS" in the publication, "Is human ageing still mysterious enough to be left only to scientists?" (de Grey et al. 2002). He later used "SENS" (as the full acronym) in the publication, "Time to talk SENS: critiquing the immutability of human ageing" (de Grey et al. 2002).

But perhaps the most significant publication in terms of a reaching wider public audience (as opposed to mainstream academic journals) was the one about Aubrey and de Grey and SENS that was authored by Sherwin Nuland (February, 2005) in *MIT Technology Review.* In our opinion, it was soon after this publication that the firestorm of controversy on slowing the ageing process, on reversing the ageing process, on anti-ageing medicine, on post ageing, on posthumanism and transhumanism, and on the role of biotechnology in the ageing process began in earnest within both the academic domain and throughout the mass media. Nuland's (2005) article in *MIT Technology Review* not only had the intriguing title of, "Do You Want To Live Forever," but it also had de Grey's bearded face gracing the entire front cover along with the more provocative headline of, "Live Forever? Aubrey de Grey Thinks He Can Defeat Death. Is He Nuts?" Although Nuland (2005) who passed away in March of 2014, went on record to indicate that he had "no desire to live beyond the life span that nature has granted to our species" he did make it clear he was in support of the notion of compression of morbidity and sounded in fact very much in favor of the optimization of ageing. Nuland (2005) also acknowledged the role that de Grey had taken on as the leading spokesperson for "anti-ageing" and for being at the right time and place in history,

> His [Aubrey de Grey] tireless efforts at thrusting himself and his theories into the vanguard of a movement in pursuit of a goal of eternal fascination to the human mind have put him among the most prominent proponents of antiaging science in the world. His timing is perfect. As the baby boomers—perhaps the most determinedly self-improving (and self-absorbed) generation in history—are now approaching or have reached their early 60 s, there is a plenitude of eager seekers after the death-defiant panaceas he promises. de Grey has become more than a man; he is a movement. (p. 40)

Nuland's (2005) article also revealed (through the lens of Nuland's perspective) the personality, the attitudes, the values and the ethical stance of de Grey on developing SENS and extending life beyond—*way beyond*—the current assumptions of maximum life span. Here are some excerpts from the article,

> de Grey:
> The reason we have an imperative, we have a duty, to develop these therapies as soon as possible is to give future generations the choice. People are entitled, have a human right, to live as long as they can…as they want to…the right to live as long as you choose is the world's most fundamental right…This seems to be something that all moral codes, religious or secular, seem to agree on: that the right to life is the most important right…It's

not a question of how long life should be, but whether the end of life should be hastened by action or inaction.

Nuland:
And there it is—the ultimate leap of ingenious argumentation that would do a sophist proud: by our inaction in not pursuing the possible opportunity of extending life for thousands of years, we are hastening death.

In our opinion, Nuland's (2005) article was also the flame that lit the fuse on an explosion of perspectives and debate that then created an avalanche of writings to follow. In large part, we think it had to do with Nuland's style of writing, which blended both admiration and trepidation over the possibility that de Grey might actually succeed at his "benevolent" goals of extending human life, but at the same time unleash some sort of "hell scenario" (a la Garreau 2005) due to some "unanticipated havoc at both the cellular and societal level" (Nuland 2005, p. 45). In other words, Nuland was dubious about de Grey's chances to succeed (but still admired his dedication to the challenge) and was furthermore philosophically skeptical about those (like de Grey) who would seek to break the "natural" limit set for life span of humans and whether or not "it is a good thing for men and women now populating the earth to have the means to live indefinitely" (p. 42). But Nuland (2005) was not alone in being skeptical and concerned about de Grey's ambitions—and science. But that did not stop de Grey from pushing his agenda and rationale, and the friction and factions continued to escalate.

In July, 2005 de Grey published an article, "Resistance to debate on how to postpone ageing is delaying progress and costing lives" in *European Molecular Biology Organization (EMBO) Reports,* which critiqued the "rhetoric" of mainstream biogerontologists in their dealings with policy makers and the public. de Grey (2005a) took exception to the prevailing view in biogerontology with its emphasis that (1) ageing is not a disease, (2) the focus on compression of morbidity is the goal of biomedical gerontology, and (3) the potential for late-onset calorie restriction mimetics to postpone human ageing should be highlighted. de Grey also criticized the community's reluctance to engage in open-minded public scrutiny of novel approaches to postponing ageing, especially his SENS (Strategies for Engineered Negligible Senescence) proposal. The essay by de Grey (2005a) then led to strong rejoinder by a large group of "mainstream" biogerontologists (including Jay Olshansky, Bruce Carnes, and Thomas Perls) in November, 2005 with the article, "Science fact and the SENS agenda" (Warner et al. 2005) launched a scathing counterattack by claiming that none of the SENS activities has been shown to "extend the lifespan of any organism, let alone humans" and labeled de Grey's work as a "farrago" and all but dismissed it as "science fiction." de Grey (2005b) responded, "Like it or not, life-extension research extends beyond biogerontology" by emphasizing the differences in the approach of *technology* versus *science* and the narrow-mindedness of "mainstream" biogerontologists. de Grey (2005b) noted that,

Warner *and colleagues* are avowedly in the business of saving lives, just like me; dogma must not obstruct our common cause. They do not challenge my arguments that adherence to biologically and politically naive rhetoric is precisely why gerontology continues to have such trouble impressing policy-makers, yet they steadfastly defend that rhetoric as if somehow one more push will change everything. I offer no apology for using media interest in life extension to make the biology of ageing an exception to Planck's observation that science advances funeral by funeral: lives, lots of them, are at stake. (p. 1000)

So in a sense, the polarization had begun within the ranks of biogerontology (see Gray and Bürkle 2006) and de Grey (2006a) continued to defend and elaborate on his Strategies for Engineered Negligible Senescence (SENS) by indicating its differences in methodology from mainstream biogerontology and why the "compression of morbidity" is lacking in efficacy compared to the promise of SENS (see also de Grey 2006b). In other words, de Grey challenged the "dogma" of biogerontology and argued for a new way to conduct the process by which ageing would be defeated and which would lead to four-digit life spans in people alive today. The escalation of the challenge continued in several outlets like *The Chronicle of Higher Education* (see de Grey 2006c, "A Controversial Theory About Ageing") and with the announcement of a $20,000 prize by *Technology Review* (in 2005) to determine if de Grey's SENS was "so wrong that it was not worthy of learned debate." Several submissions were submitted to challenge de Grey's anti-ageing proposals and in the end, the judges determined that,

SENS is a collection of hypotheses that have mostly not been subjected to that process [the scientific process] and thus cannot rise to the level of being scientifically verified. However, by the same token, the ideas of SENS have not been conclusively disproved. SENS exists in a middle ground of yet-to-be-tested ideas that some people may find intriguing but which others are free to doubt. (*Technology Review*, July/August, 2006, p. 80).

But de Grey (2006d) saw the declaration of a "tie" (or that the fact that *no submission* met the criterion of the challenge and disproved SENS) as a "win" and called upon the field to "get back to work." Further editorials by de Grey followed, as well as counterarguments by others (see Warner 2006), predominantly in the journal *Rejuvenation Research* (see Warner 2006) that kept the battle engaged. By 2006, it became clear that Aubrey de Grey's SENS proposal was going to sustain itself in the literature, in the headlines for popular magazines, and on the Internet due to the sheer tenacity and relentless presentation format delivered by de Grey. de Grey obviously relished the debates with professionals in both gerontology and geriatrics and the ongoing dialogue as it continued to bring attention to the SENS project and the way in which it differed from the tenets of mainstream biogerontology (or gerontology for that matter) as he challenged the received view and marked the difference between scientific and technological progress. But, the culmination of those efforts resulted in the publication, *Ending Ageing:The Rejuvenation Breakthroughs That Could Reverse Human Ageing in Our Lifetime* (de Grey and Rae 2007) designed for the mass market. In this book, de Grey compares his battle to defeat ageing akin to the public health campaign to eliminate smoking,

> Yet, in the sense that matters most, ageing is just like smoking: It's really bad for you. It shortens your life, it typically makes the last several years of your life rather grim, and it also makes those years pretty hard on your loved ones. (p. 10)

de Grey and Rae (2007) also proffered an interesting theory about the motivations for the "pro-ageing trance" that appears to have a grip on people's attitudes and fear (of ending ageing); he claims it has little to do with the usual suspects—the specter of overpopulation or that only the wealthy elite would enjoy the benefits of maximum life extension (or immortality)—but rather that it is based in the existential surrender of any hope for anything different than what is our supposed destiny of a "limited" life span for *Homo sapiens*. de Grey explained that until recently, ageing has been inescapable, and so the easiest, most effective way for people to cope is to simply ignore it.

Yet, de Grey is preoccupied with defeating ageing, and sees little benefit or reward, even if optimization were to take place or morbidity were compressed in experiencing the ageing process as it simply represents a Hobbesian nightmare (i.e., "the life of man, solitary, poor, nasty, brutish, and short") that needs to be changed, modified, and modulated as though ageing were a *disease*. And all of this begs the question of *how*—how would de Grey go about eliminating ageing from the human life course?

Let's assume that such a project and campaign to end ageing would take a lot of research funding; de Grey is up front with this critical condition and has co-founded *The Methuselah Foundation* (http://www.methuselahfoundation.org) as an attempt to address that issue (see also the Manhattan Beach Project, http://www.manhattanbeachproject.com). But again, the focus of this book is on the role of technology in the post ageing inflection point, especially in the radical version [5.5 and >], so de Grey's proposals are very much centered around a technological interventionist approach (via SENS) based on *engineering rejuvenation*, relying on coming technological advances to amplify the outcomes toward longevity escape velocity (LEV). de Grey and Rae (2007) was also very adamant about how SENS differs from *geriatrics* (which also uses medical technology; see also Callahan 2009; Reiser 2009) and *gerontological* (which also uses technology) approaches to the ageing process and one of the key differences among them is *when* the technology is used to intervene with the process of ageing.

> Might it be possible to repair damage after it's been laid down (hence avoiding the need to understand the details of how it's laid down) but spirals out of control (hence also avoiding the losing battle that is geriatrics)? (p. 41)

The point taken from de Grey's perspective here is that the traditional approaches in using technologies in the context of the study of ageing have been *too early* ("over-preemptive") by "simply" trying to understand and discover metabolic processes at the cellular level (without repairing accumulating damage), or *too late* in the use of medical interventions via geriatric medicine ("a losing battle") or *too little* by using technologies in the assistive dimension (what our heuristic would consider *moderate* versions) which are interventions primarily *external* to the individual such as modifications to the physical environment (e.g., the residential setting of the older adult), the use of computers to monitor the various measures of health status for older adults, or the use of the internet for information access. In effect, de Grey and Rae 2007) was proposing the more radical step of repairing damage "in the sweet spot" of intervention (not through traditional gerontological and geriatric approaches), directly to the source of the "ageing" (cellular and molecular), by using current and (assumed) near future technological advances (e.g., nanomedicine—see Schulz et al. 2009) to manipulate the process of senescence. Furthermore, de Grey and Rae (2007) leaves behind the constraints of the traditional scientific model and brings (especially if scholars embrace the notion of interdisciplinarity in the study of ageing) a new approach, a new vision, for addressing the negative consequences of senescence. Notice we said "negative" consequences, since de Grey appears to find little (or no) redeeming consequences in experiencing the natural process of ageing. Rather, for de Grey, ageing is comprehensively an "all or nothing" conceptualization; there is no compressing of morbidity nor is ageing seen as a fertile ground for Stoic reflection or existential contemplation—no, ageing is to be lifted out of the socially-constructed and the philosophically-minded halls of academe and into a highly developed "repair shop" to fix the flawed metabolic, carbon-based, multi-cellular, bi-pedal, and neocortical unit that is known as *Homo sapiens*—so that it does not have to face the ageing process at all:

> You could stop thinking of ageing as a hopelessly *theoretical* problem to solve, and get on with attacking it head-on, as an *engineering challenge* that needed to be overcome. (p. 44)

Obviously, de Grey thinks the key—and solution to the problem—is to use engineering and technological interventions to end ageing—*period*. There is no need to discuss metaphysics, theories, and necessarily ethics; rather, the goal is to produce *results* by changing the nature of *what is*—to manipulate nature for the betterment of the human life experience so that ageing itself is never realized. Thus, post ageing, or beyond ageing, or ageing to be known only as an artifact—as something that once was; in the future, ageing is *not to be*.

But of course this orientation to the ageing experience and process is not without its critics from a biodemography and biogerontology perspective (Olshansky et al. 2004) within evolutionary biology (Rose 2005, 2009), and ethical perspectives (Muller 2007; Lucke et al. 2009; Underwood et al. 2009; Temkin 2008). Nevertheless, de Grey (2009a) is intent on razing the "pro-ageing edifice" that is the dominant view of many bio- and social gerontologists who embrace a "compression of morbidity" or "optimization of ageing" or "disease management" (see Jackson and Bartek 2009), but then decline to entertain the possibility of life extension beyond the "natural" maximum life span. These "pro-ageing" scientists allegedly see no value or efficacy in *engineering rejuvenation* because it does fit into either the "received view" of gerontology and geriatrics and, as any other "paradigm" outside of mainstream scientific methodology, is deemed "pseudo-science." This is a critical issue for any potential success in the implementation of SENS as de Grey (2009b) has claimed that scientists within traditional gerontology and geriatrics are misunderstanding the role of technology versus the activities of science,

> In science, the objective is to discover the way world works, whereas in technology, the objective is to exploit science to change how things work. Science is ultimately about predicting nature, while technology is about manipulating nature. (p. 75)

Another way to describe the difference in approach (and attitudes) toward investigating the ageing process versus "fixing" it is with the following metaphor of "roof repair" for a decrepit house.

> The man on the ground is a gerontologist—digging to see if the tree roots are undermining the house foundations (causes). The man on the step-ladder is a geriatrician—mending the house ceiling (symptoms), and the engineer on the roof—repairing and containing the damage as he goes along. This is the de Grey engineering approach to 'ending ageing.' (Spurling 2009, p. 24.)

As the debate continues, it is no surprise that "outsider" journalist/blogger/writers like Critser (2010), *Eternity Soup: Inside the Quest to End Ageing*, Stipp (2010), *The Youth Pill: Scientists at the Brink of an Anti-Ageing Revolution*, and Weiner (2010), *Long for This World: The Strange Science of Immortality*, would enter the fray by reviewing the developments in the field and the characters who are involved, taking sides on the various issues of post ageing. Critser (2010) took the angle of the objective, yet curious, innocent pilgrim who enters into a strange land for the first time, marveling at the shape-shifting science and medicine of *longevity*, which appears to be a cacophony of characters, concepts, and contradictions that could, ultimately, make a good story to write about in his investigative sojourn into the land of Big G and Little G (Critser 2010). According to Critser, Big G represents many (not all) of us who are members of the Gerontological Society of America (GSA), reading this journal, the *Journals of Gerontology*, and *The Gerontologist.* Big G supposedly represents the "gerontology establishment" who follow the marching orders of our dogmatic and received view without question. That is, there appears to be an agenda—hidden or otherwise, that we are following and have allegiance to. And the area of "science" where Critser believes the battle lines have been drawn is in the domain of anti-ageing research ("longevity medicine", or life span extension) because it is those within the Little G camp (as seen by the Big G group) who carry out their rebellious quest, rogue operations, and counterfactual strategies to challenge the dogma and the status quo of the Big G group. In other words, the skirmishes between Big G and Little G over the quest to end ageing are more than just loyalty and identification with the array of possible interventions (e.g., caloric restriction, resveratrol, human growth hormone, antioxidants, genetic engineering, and biotechnologies), or debating the nuances and extrapolations of research on rodents to humans; there is something bigger at stake here. From Critser's vantage point, it is how, and why, the entire enterprise of science should proceed to address the ageing experience, and whether or not ageing is even something that needs to be manipulated and eradicated. Depending on one's perspective, Big G is defending "science" and guarding against the quackery, charlatans, and pseudo scientists (or a "farrago" as de Grey

2006a, calls it) that some associate with the Little G camp. From another perspective, the Little G camp is portrayed as the creative and heroic David searching for new solutions against the mighty Goliath (notice the big "G"), tyrannical in protecting its turf and bent on hurling pretentious diatribes against those (in the Little G camp) who go against the grain of tradition and protocol. And there is much at stake with image, marketing, policy, and of course money, both in research funding and in the profits from selling goods to a ready and willing "paying" public. Critser (2010) proposed that,

> The longer I mingled with anti-ageing types, both those with traditional degrees and those without, the more I came to appreciate the reason Big G hates them. It is this: They are surfing on—and making money from—the establishment's science, long before scientists—and most of the time, even ordinary folk—would deem science sufficient...Big G has little faith that such pseudoscience will debunk itself. They may be right. If anything, the marketing is slicker and more even soaked in science (p. 105).

But many of those in the Little G Camp, like de Grey (2009c), spend a great deal of energy breaking the "pro-ageing edifice" that is the domain and prevailing view of many bio- and social gerontologists who embrace a "compression of morbidity", "optimization of ageing", or "disease management" (see Jackson and Bartek 2009), but refuse to entertain the possibility of life extension beyond the "natural" maximum life span.

A similar kind of reporting style (and investigation) is found in Weiner's (2010) book, *Long for this World: The Strange Science of Immortality*. Weiner (2010) also takes the long view by placing the quest to "end ageing" in a historical and interdisciplinary perspective. And similar to Critser (2010), he discovered that while the field of gerontology is in the midst of incredible excitement due to developments in bioengineering and technology, the "...field is so splintered and spiky right now that it's hard to find a majority view. Gerontologists can't agree on a way to measure ageing, or what they mean by ageing" (p. 15).

Weintraub (2010) took a different perspective with her investigative reporting in her book, *Selling the Fountain of Youth: How the Anti-Ageing Industry Made a Disease Out of Getting Old—And Made Billions.* As one can ascertain from the title, Weintraub (2010) skewers the "longevity industry" and takes exception to the notion that ageing is a disease. She was especially critical of hormonal treatments as basically useless and potentially dangerous as a supposed intervention.

Perhaps the ultimate indicator of the intersect of science, Big G and little G, and the media exemplar for post ageing would be the documentary film (available on DVD) which takes the existential dilemma of Hamlet and wraps it into a modern day gerontological docu-drama titled, *To Age or Not To Age*: *That is the Question*, a film by Pappas (2010). We have entered into the post ageing era when it is possible to ask (both rhetorically and in actuality) whether to age or not age– and that is *the* (a la Shakespeare) question for our time. And this perspective, this new paradigm, this new inflection point, we believe will bring us, ultimately, right back to the beginning—the philosophy of ageing.

References

Aaron, H. J., & Schwartz, W. B. (Eds.). (2004). *Coping with methuselah*. Washington, DC: Brookings Institution Press.
Adams, E., Nolan, V., Andersen, S., Perls, T., & Terry, D. (2008). Centenarian offspring: Start healthier and stay healthier. *Journal of American Geriatrics Society, 56*, 2089–2092.
Adleman, R. C. (1995). The alzheimerization of ageing. *The Gerontologist, 35*(4), 526–532.
Anton, T. (2013). *The longevity seekers: Science, business, and the fountain of youth*. Chicago, IL: University of Chicago Press.
Atala, A., Lanza, R., Thomson, J., & Nerem, R. (Eds.). (2010). *Foundations of regenerative medicine*. San Diego, CA: Academic Press (Elsevier).
Baudisch, A. (2008). *Inevitable ageing? Contributions to evolutionary-demographic theory*. Berlin, Germany: Springer.
Binstock, R. (2003). The war on 'anti-ageing medicine'. *The Gerontologist, 43*(1), 4–14.
Binstock, R. H. (2004). Anti-ageing medicine and research: A realm of conflict and profound societal implications. *Journals of Gerontology: Biological Sciences and Medical Sciences, 59A*(6), 523.
Brey, P. (2009). Human enhancement and personal identity. In J. Olsen, E. Selinger, & S. Riss (Eds.), *New waves in philosophy of technology* (pp. 169–185). New York: Palgrave Macmillan.
Callahan, D. (Ed.). (2009). *Taming the beloved beast: How medical technology costs are destroying our health care system*. Princeton, NJ: Princeton University Press.
Carnes, B., & Olshansky, S. J. (2007). A realist view of ageing, mortality, and future longevity. *Population and Development Review, 33*(2), 367–381.
Comfort, A. (1964). *The Ageing of Senescence*. New York: Holt, Rinehart and Winston, Inc. (first published in 1956 as *The Biology of Senescence*).
Critser, G. (2010). *Eternity soup: Inside the quest to end ageing*. New York: Harmony Books.
de Grey, A. D. N. J. (2004). Escape velocity: Why the prospect of extreme human life extension matters now. *PLoS Biology, 2*(6), 0723–0726.
de Grey, A. D. N. J. (2005a). Resistance to debate on how to postpone ageing is delaying progress and costing lives. *EMBO Reports, 6*, S49–S53.
de Grey, A. D. N. J. (2005b). Like or not, life extension research extends beyond biogerontology. *EMBO Reports, 6*, 1000.
de Grey, A. D. N. J. (2006a). Is SENS a farrago? *Rejuvenation Research, 9*(4), 436–439.
de Grey, A. D. N. J. (2006b). Compression of morbidity: The hype and the reality, part 1. *Rejuvenation Research, 9*(1), 1–2.
de Grey, A. D. N. J. (2006c). A controversial theory about ageing (Letter to the editor). *The Chronicle of Higher Education, 52*(18), A63.
de Grey, A. D. N. J. (2009a). Cracks in social gerontology's pro-ageing edifice. *Rejuvenation Research, 12*(1), 1–2.
de Grey, A. D. N. J. (2009b). The curiously misunderstood role of evidence in designing new technology. *Rejuvenation Research, 12*, 75.
de Grey, A. D. N. J. (2009c). The singularity and the methuselarity: Similarities and differences. *Studies in Health Technology and Informatics, 149*, 195–202.
de Grey, A. D. N. J. (2006d). SENS survives the challenge: Now let's get back to work. *Rejuvenation Research, 9*(4), 429–430.
de Grey, A. D. N. J., Ames, B., Andersen, J., Bartke, A., Campisi, J., Heward, C., et al. (2002a). Time to talk SENS: Critiquing the immutability of human ageing. *Annals of New York Academy of Science, 942*, 452–462.
de Grey, A. D. N. J., Baynes, J.W., Berd, J., Heward, C.B. Graham Pawelec, G., & Stock, G. (2002). Is human ageing still mysterious enough to be left only to scientists? *BioEssays 24*, 667–676.

de Grey, A. D. N. J., & Rae, M. (2007). *Ending ageing: The rejuvenation breakthrough that could reverse human ageing in our Lifetime*. New York: St. Martin's Press.

DeLashmutt, M. W. (2006). A better life through information technology? The techno-theological eschatology of posthuman speculative science {Perspectives on techno-science and human nature}. *Zygon, 41*, 267–287.

Dodd, S. B. (1921). *Old age: Its cause and prevention*. New York: Mead & Co.

Estes, C. (1993). The ageing enterprise revisited. *The Gerontologist, 33*(3), 292–297.

Fishman, J. R., Binstock, R. H., & Lambrix, M. A. (2008). Anti-ageing science: The emergence, maintenance, and enhancement of a discipline. *Journal of Ageing Studies, 22*, 295–303.

Fukuyama, F. (2002). *Our posthuman future: Consequences of the biotechnology revolution*. New York: Farrar, Straus and Giroux.

Garreau, J. (2005). *Radical evolution: The promise and peril of enhancing our minds, our bodies—and what it means to be human*. New York: Broadway (Random House.

General Accountability Office. (2001). *Health products for seniors: "Anti-ageing" products pose potential for physical and economic harm,* GAO-01-1129. http://www.gao.gov/products/GAO-01-1139T.

Goldsmith, T. C. (2008). Ageing, evolvability, and the individual benefit requirement; medical implications of ageing theory controversies. *Journal of Theoretical Biology, 252*, 764–768.

Goldman, D. P., Cutler, D., Rowe, J. W., Michaud, P. C., Sullivan, J., Peneva, D., et al. (2013). Substantial health and economic returns from delayed ageing may warrant a new focus for medical research. *Health Affairs, 32*(10), 1698–1705.

Gray, D. A., & Bürkle, A. (2006). SENS and the polarization of ageing-related research. *Science of Ageing Knowledge Environment* April (7). http://sageke.sciencemag.org/cgi/content/full/2006/7/pe8.

Haber, C. (2004). Life extension and history: The continual search for the fountain of youth. *Journal of Gerontology: Biological Sciences, 59A*(6), 515–522.

Hadley, E., Lakatta, E., Morrison-Bogorad, M., Warner, H., & Hodes, R. (2005). The future of ageing therapies. *Cell, 120*(4), 557–567.

Hall, S. G. (1922). *Senescence: The last half of life*. New York: D. Appleton & Co.

Hall, S. S. (2003). *Merchants of immortality: Chasing the dream of human life extension*. New York: Houghton Mifflin.

Hall, W. J. (2008). Centenarians: Metaphor becomes reality. *Archives of Internal Medicine, 168*(3), 262–263.

Hayflick, L. (1994). *How and why we age*. New York: Ballantine Books.

Hayflick, L. (2004). "Anti-ageing" is an oxymoron. *Journal of Gerontology: BIOLOGICAL SCIENCES, 59A*(6), 573–578.

Hayflick, L. (2009). *Ageing is so longer an unsolved biological problem*. Paper presented at the World Congress of Gerontology and Geriatrics, Paris, France.

Hildt, E. (2009). Living longer: Age retardation and autonomy. *Medical Health Care and Philosophy, 12*, 179–185.

Jackson, S. P., & Bartek, J. (2009). The DNA-damage response in human biology and disease. *Nature, 461*, 1071–1078.

Joyce, K., & Loe, M. (2009). A sociological approach to ageing, technology and health. *Sociology of Health & Illness, 32*(2), 171–180.

Kampf, A., & Botelho, L. A. (2009). Anti-ageing and biomedicine: Critical studies on the pursuit of maintaining, revitalizing and enhancing ageing bodies. *Medicine Studies, 1*, 187–195.

Kurzweil, R. (2009). Ray Kurzweil on how to combat ageing. *MIT Technology Review*. http://www.technologyreview.com/view/414240/ray-kurzweil-on-how-to-combat-ageing/.

Kurzweil, R., & Grossman, T. (2009). *Transcend: Nine steps to living well forever*. New York: Rodale.

Martin, G. (2006). Keynote lecture: An update on the what, why, and how questions of ageing. *Experimental Gerontology, 41*, 460–463.

Michel, J., Newton, J., & Kirkwood, T. (2008). Medical challenges of improving the quality of a longer life. *JAMA, 299*(6), 688–690.

Mittledorf, J., & Pepper, J. (2009). Senescence as an adaption to limit the spread of disease. *Journal of Theoretical Biology* (Sept.), *260*, 186–195.

Muller, F. S. (2007). On futuristic gerontology: A philosophical evaluation of Aubrey de Grey's SENS Project. *International Journal of Applied Philosophy, 21*(2), 225–239.

Mykytyn, C. E. (2006a). Anti-ageing medicine: A patient/practitioner movement to redefine ageing. *Social Science and Medicine, 62*, 643–653.

Mykytyn, C. E. (2006b). Anti-ageing medicine: Predictions, moral obligations, and biomedical intervention. *Anthropological Quarterly, 79*(1), 5–31.

Mykytyn, C. (2008). Medicalizing the optimal: Anti-ageing medicine and the quandary. *Journal of Ageing Studies, 22*, 313–321.

Norris, S., High, K., Gill, T., Hennessy, S., Kutner, J., Reuben, D., et al. (2008). Health care for Older Americans with multiple chronic conditions: A research agenda. *Journal of Americans Geriatrics Society, 56*, 149.

Nuland, S. B. (2005, February). Do you want to live forever? *MIT Technology Review*. http://www.technologyreview.com/featuredstory/403654/do-you-want-to-live-forever/.

Olshansky, S. J. (1998). On the biodemography of ageing: A review essay. *Population and Development Review (24)*2, 381-393.

Olshansky, S. J., & Carnes, B. (2001). *The quest for immortality: Science at the frontiers of ageing*. New York: W.W. Norton & Co.

Olshansky, S. J., & Carnes, B. A. (2009). The future of longevity. In P. Uhlenberg (Ed.), *International handbook of population ageing* (pp. 731–745). New York: Springer.

Olshansky, S. J., Hayflick, L., & Carnes, B. (2002a). No truth to the fountain of youth. *Scientific American, 286*(6), 92–95.

Olshansky, S. J., Hayflick, L., & Carnes, B. (2002b). Position statement on human ageing. *Journal of Gerontology: Biological Science, 57A*(8), B292–B297.

Olshansky, S. J., Hayflick, L., & Perls, T. (2004). Anti-ageing medicine: The hype and the reality—Part I. *Journal of Gerontology: BIOLOGICAL SCIENCES, 59A*(6), 513–514.

Pappas, R. L. (2010). *To age or not to age: That is the question*. Sag Harbor Basement Pictures [DVD].

Partridge, B., Lucke, J., & Hall, W. (2009a). Ethical, social, and personal implications of extended human lifespan identified by members of the public. *Rejuvenation Research, 12*(5), 351–357.

Partridge, B., Underwood, M., Lucke, J., Bartlett, H., & Hall, W. (2009b). Ethical concerns in the community about technologies to extend human life span. *The American Journal of Bioethics, 9*(12), 68–76.

Perls, T., Kohler, I. V., Andersen, S., Schoenhofen, E., Pennington, J., Young, R., et al. (2007). Survival of parents and siblings of supercentenarians. *Journal of Gerontology: Medical Sciences, 62A*, 1028–1034.

Post, S. (2004). Establishing an appropriate ethical framework: The moral conversation around the goal of prolongevity. *Journals of Gerontology. Series A, Biological Sciences and Medical Sciences, 59*(6), B534–B539.

Reiser, S. J. (2009). *Technological medicine: The changing world of doctors and patients*. New York: Cambridge University Press.

Reuben, D. B. (2007). Update in geriatric medicine. *Annals of Intgernal Medicine, 147*(7), 470–477.

Robine, J. M., Crimmins, E., Horiuchi, S., & Yi, Z. (Eds.). (2006). *Human longevity, individual life duration, and the growth of the oldest-old population*. Dordrecht, The Netherlands: Springer.

Rose, M. R. (2005). *The long tomorrow: How advances in evolutionary biology can help us postpone ageing*. New York: Oxford University Press.

Rose, M. R. (2009). Adaptation, ageing, and genomic information. *Ageing, 1*(5), 444–450.

Schulz, M. J., Shanov, V. N., & Yun, Y. (2009). *Nanomedicine; Design of particles, sensors, motors, implants, robots, and devices*. Boston, MA: Artech House.

Spurling, A. (2009). The end of ageing? *Engineering & Technology, 14* (March/April), 22–25.

Stipp, D. (2010). *The youth pill: Scientists at the brink of an anti-ageing revolution*. New York: Current (Penguin).

Stock, G., & Callahan, D. (2004) Point–counterpoint: Would doubling the human life span be a net positive or negative for us either as individuals or as a society? *Journals of GerontologySeries A Biological Sciences and Medical Sciences 59*(A), 554.

Temkin, L. S. (2008). Is living longer living better? *Journal of Applied Philosophy, 25*(3), 193–210.

Turner, L. (2004). Biotechnology, bioethics, and antiageing interventions. *Trends in Biotechnology, 22*(5), 219–221.

Vina, J., Borras, C., & Miquel, J. (2007). Theories of ageing. *International Union of Biochemistry and Molecular Biology Life, 59*(4–5), 249–254.

Vincent, J. (2003). What is at stake in the 'war on anti-ageing medicine'? *Ageing and Society, 23*, 675–684.

Vincent, J. (2006). Ageing contested: Anti-ageing science and the cultural construction of old age. *Sociology, 40*(4), 681–698.

Vincent, J. (2008). The cultural construction old age as a biological phenomenon: Science and anti-ageing technologies. *Journal of Ageing Studies, 22*, 331–339.

Vincent, J., Tulle, E., & Bond, J. (2008). The anti-ageing enterprise: Science, knowledge, expertise, rhetoric and values. *Journal of Ageing Studies, 22*, 291–294.

Wachter, K. W., & Finch, C. (1997). *Between Zeus and the salmon: the biodemography of longevity*. Washington, DC: National Academy Press.

Warner, H. R. (2006). Scientific and ethical concerns regarding engineering human longevity. *Rejuvenation Research, 9*(4), 440–442.

Warner, H., Anderson, J., Austad, S., Bergamini, E., Bredesen, D., Butler, R., et al. (2005). Science fact and the SENS agenda: What can we reasonably expect from ageing research? *EMBO Reports, 6*, 1006–1008.

Warthin, A. S. (1930). *Old age: The major involution: The physiology and pathology of the ageing process*. New York: Paul B. Hoeber Inc.

Weiner, J. (2010). *Long for this world: The strange science of immortality*. New York: HarperCollins.

Weintraub, A. (2010). *Selling the fountain of youth: How the anti-ageing industry made a disease out of getting old-and made billions*. New York: Basic Books.

Wright, S. D. (2008). Life in the long lane—a review essay on the longevity revolution: The benefits and challenges of living a long lifeby Robert N. Butler. *Journal of the American Heart Association* 2(3/4), 298–313.

Yates, L. Djousse, L., Kurth, T., Buring, J., & Gaziano, M. (2008). Exceptional longevity in men: Modifiable factors associated with survival and function to age 90 years. *Archives of Internal Medicine, 168*(3), 284–290.

Zs-Nagy, I. (2009). Is consensus in anti-ageing medical intervention an elusive expectation or a realistic goal? *Archives of Gerontology and Geriatrics, 48*, 271–275.

Chapter 7
Viable Criticisms for the Radical Version of Post Ageing [5.5 and >]

Abstract The radical version of the "post ageing" inflection point (and its exemplars) is simply not satisfied with scientific advancements to merely compress morbidity, know about the causes of the how and why of ageing, optimize ageing, or to manipulate and modify only the external environments that surround the ageing individual (e.g., assistive technology)—no, the goals are more monumental with dramatic consequences for just about every sphere of human existence. In our opinion, at the very core of the motivation and operations of SENS, and SENSE, and the possibility of a technological singularity (see Goertzel 2007; Kurzweil 2005) is to move beyond ageing so that the *modus operandi* in the radical version is to modify, rejuvenate, and transcend (see Harris 2010). The goal is not to simply make the best of what we have, rather it is to make more—and better—than what we have (Garreau 2005). The radical version of post ageing will only be satisfied when scientific advancements and the use of technologies can fully intervene with the internal environment of the human body and address the ultimate "limits" of human finitude and uniqueness (the epitome of intelligence). Indeed, it is the specter of mortality, the presence of death as a natural outcome of human existence that is to be reckoned with assertively, and most decisively through SENS, SENSE, and Singularity.

Keywords Bioconservative · Etiology of ageing · Evolutionary biology · Methuselarity · Radical human lifespan extension · SENS · SENSE · Singularity · Technoprogressive

The disparagements against this approach are two-fold, and fall under the categories of evolutionary biology and philosophy/metaphysics.

7.1 Evolutionary Biology

As mentioned previously, the bioengineering approach (i.e., SENS) as a viable intervention to "cure ageing" has received substantive critique from biodemographers and biogerontologists. SENS has been labeled as "non-scientific", or has

K.F. Felsted and S.D. Wright, *Toward Post Ageing*,
Healthy Ageing and Longevity 1, DOI 10.1007/978-3-319-09051-1_7

been vested with little confidence as a promise of rejuvenation engineering, or has wilted in the face of the fundamental belief that radical life extension is simply not going to happen (see Critser 2010; Stipp 2010; Weiner 2010). This is exemplified in the Medical Life Expectancy Debate with Aubrey de Grey and S. Jay Olshansky at the 2nd Life Settlements and Longevity Summit (September 30–October 1 2009; New York, NY) where de Grey and Olshansky had to address the fundamental question: Is radical human lifespan extension within our grasp? de Grey argued for and Olshansky against the motion and both went on record (via the news release from the conference organizers, http://www.lifesettlementsummit.com) to state that,

> "Radical postponement of age-related ill-health is a feasible medical goal." de Grey argued that there is a 50 % chance of life extension therapies arriving in 25–30 years. If that happens, life spans could theoretically be extended almost indefinitely and it's possible that the first person to live for a thousand years is actually alive today.

Dr. S. Jay Olshansky, on the other hand, makes the case that radical life extension is not going to happen—if it ever happens—in time to influence any of the investment decisions made by those involved with life settlements or insurance linked securities. Olshansky continues, "Nothing in gerontology comes close to fulfilling the promise of dramatically extended human lifespans, but it may soon be possible to slow ageing enough to influence Institutional Life Settlements (ILS) in the near-term."

While the debate between de Grey and Olshansky appears to be based on mutual respect, there is still deep disagreement regarding the fundamentals of how "science" is conducted and whether there is viability in manipulating nature to extend life beyond the "natural" limit. But I think there are also larger contentious issues that serve as undercurrents to the whole debate of SENS, life extension, and the possibility of immortality. For example, de Grey symbolically represents either a Dr. Frankenstein/Faust figure, or an heroic "outsider"—the maverick willing to take on the established mainstream of biogerontology and biodemography, moving quickly to the forefront of media attention. He also has assertively pushed back against the collective brain trust of professional groups (whom he calls the "pro-ageing edifice") in gerontology and geriatrics with relentless rebuttals and counterattacks. In addition to the perceived siphoning of media attention and recognition away from "legitimate" scientific projects on the biology of ageing, and toward de Grey (with his eccentric appearance and provocative claims) and his SENS project, there is the audacious requesting of funds in a direct appeal the public and philanthropic foundations to The Methuselah Foundation.

Also, as previously mentioned, there were the critiques from evolutionary biology (Rose 2005, 2008) and from an ethical perspective (Muller 2007).The evolutionary biological perspective of ageing has an interesting history that can be traced back to a paper by Hamilton (1966), "The Moulding of Senescence by Natural Selection," and according to Rose et al. (2007), it was then that Hamilton, in 1966, provided an overarching framework for understanding the power of natural selection at early ages, the existence of ageing, the timing of ageing, the cessation of ageing, and the timing of the cessation of ageing (see also Bourke 2007; Ljubuncic and Reznick 2009). However, the literature has indicated several challenges to the Hamiltonian perspective (see Martin 2005), but Martin (2006) still sees the evolutionary biological theory of why we age as the "best game in town." Yet as the field matures and expands some have wondered if the current understanding of ageing (from a genetic and evolutionary biological perspective) is clouded because of key terms used to describe genetic effects, such as "regulation of lifespan" or "regulation of ageing" (Lithgow 2006). Nevertheless, there continue to be provocative perspectives on ageing that surface in the field of evolutionary biology discussing the "function" and purpose of ageing and the prospects for medical intervention in the ageing process (Sell et al. 2009). For example, Goldsmith (2008) examined the class of theories of ageing known as adaptive ageing (a.k.a. ageing by design, ageing selected for its own sake, programmed death theories) and noted that these theories have enjoyed a resurgence of popularity because of the discovery of genes that promote ageing in various organisms. But then, as Goldsmith (2008) aptly pointed out, this supposedly flies in the face of traditional evolutionary theory that has postulated that it is impossible for an organism to acquire a design that produces a net reduction in individual benefit (life span of reproductive capacity) (see also Partridge and Gems 2006). But Goldsmith (2008) argued for an "adjustment" of adaptive theory of ageing ("the evolution of evolvability") which addresses the individual benefit issue and then influences the potential for medical interventions,

> For a century, ageing theory has been seen as having little practical value. Most people think that ageing is a fundamental and unavoidable process and theories based on traditional evolution mechanics tend to reinforce this belief, because they typically predict that ageing is the result of a large number of very intractable or even unalterable factors. Those that believe in genetic deterioration theories have an even dimmer view. Adaptive theories tend to be much more optimistic regarding the possibility of medical intervention in the ageing process. (p. 767–768)

Another interesting twist on the perspective of evolutionary biology and ageing was offered by Mittledorf and Pepper (2009), who examined the "motivation" for the evolution of senescence in the context of population density variations, specifically associated with famine and epidemics, that can trigger sudden population declines. Mittledorf and Pepper (2009) drew upon the theory ("the 'Red Queen' hypothesis") that sexual reproduction recombination evolved for the purpose of promoting diversity in order to protect a population from microbial epidemics, and that this same mechanism facilitates the evolution of senescence, contributing to epidemic resistance in two separate ways:

(1) Population density contributes to the transmission of disease. Senescence lowers population density by increasing the death rate; moreover it does so in a way independent of stochastic causes of mortality in the environment. Senescence at the population level can contribute to leveling the death rate in fluctuating environments.

(2) Senescence contributes to a shorter effective generation time, thereby increasing population turnover and enhancing genetic diversity.

Thus, Mittledorf and Pepper (2009) suggest that the same Red Queen mechanism that provides a powerful selective force for the evolution of sex also favors the evolution of senescence. Their perspective is an extreme theory in relation to the standard models in evolutionary biology, as it proposes that selection acts to hold population density below a threshold, which then brings with it the explanation for why there would be a direct selection of an attribute as detrimental to individual fitness as senescence or sex. Mittledorf and Pepper (2009) elaborate on the "explanation" for senescence this way,

> The mechanism proposed herein is radical in that it is outside the range of standard population genetic assumptions. But we make no claim to proffered powerful evidence; rather, the compelling evidence is in the phenomenology of ageing, which gives every evidence of being a powerful adaptation, rather than an unavoidable deterioration or a side-effect of other adaptations. Once this empirical point is recognized, we suggest that the mechanism outlined herein is among the least radical solutions to the conundrum of adaptive ageing. (p. 193)

This perspective is provocative not only for using the Red Queen hypothesis as a viable explanation for senescence as a group level adaptive strategy (from an evolutionary biological perspective; see also the "grandmother hypothesis," Hawkes et al. 1998), but it also raises the compelling question as to whether something that is recognized as "a powerful adaptation" in order to limit disease (or limit the spread of epidemics) theoretically in humans—can then be taken as the very evolutionary strategy that is then altered or manipulated via another set of strategies (i.e., SENS) put into practice by humans (see Aubrey de Grey and The Methuselah Foundation)to counter the evolutionary adaptive strategy so that the individual may circumvent senescence altogether and live longer. Which then begs another question: Does not the successful implementation of SENS add to the population density, as senescence is made negligible because of rejuvenation technologies discovered and created by humans? In other words, if you subscribe to the Red Queen hypothesis as an explanation for the adaptive strategy for senescence to evolve (in the first place) in order to limit the spread of disease, then it follows that either the human-designed SENS can seem as a disruptive and/or counterproductive intervention against what is the result of a natural selection process as a benefit for the population, or that SENS and other technological developments (such as the GRIN technologies) will enable humans to transcend the "shackles" of evolutionary biological determinants and patterns and perhaps eliminate the array of diseases that served as selection forces on Homo sapiens. In any case, the scholarly works of Rose (2005, 2008, 2009) has offered a complementary or alternative intervention strategy for postponing ageing that is based in advances in evolutionary biology—in contrast to the bioengineering approach of de Grey and SENS. A major publication by Rose (2005), *The Long Tomorrow: How Advances in Evolutionary Biology Can Help Us Postpone Ageing*, was written with both a personal and philosophical perspective to explain "how ageing is ultimately controlled by evolution, a finding that is full of promise for human welfare" (p. xi), and Rose's outlook for postponing ageing (note "postponing", not necessarily "curing" or "ending" ageing) is decidedly more optimistic than Olshansky or Hayflick.

> The basic science of ageing, especially the evolutionary biology of ageing, suggests that the postponement of human ageing would be a difficult but not impossible task for properly focused research team. The main thing lacking now is some kind of corporate setting in which such a team might work. The problem is thus more one of vision than technology. (p. 125)

Now you as the reader will note, that sounds a lot like Aubrey de Grey, but there is a key difference between evolutionary biology and the bioengineering approaches via SENS and The Methuselah Foundation and that is fully illuminated in an article by Rose (2008), "Making SENSE: Strategies for Engineering Negligible Senescence Evolutionarily" in the journal *Rejuvenation Research*. Rose (2008) is quite direct in his perspective: "only the evolutionary genetic theory of ageing provides a reasonable scientific foundation for the study or manipulation of ageing" (p. 529) and he goes further by critiquing the SENS approach in this fashion,

> Not only is it based on erroneous science, we also know enough about physiology of postponing ageing by evolutionary or dietary means to conclude that physiological mechanisms quite different from the mere accumulations of damage are extremely important. Thus a focus on damage repair is simply not going to yield negligible senescence, even it allows some mitigation of the depredations of ageing. (p. 530)

In effect, Rose (2008) argues that SENS needed to be based on re-tuning adaptation, not repairing damage. And therein lies the key differentiation. Evolutionary biology of ageing understands and predicts that there are many physiological mechanisms (not just cumulative damage) involved in the etiology of ageing and that these various mechanisms are based on adaptive strategies for the organism such that ageing may involve the allocation of resources away from somata and toward reproduction and thus the true foundation of ageing is: *a transient loss of age-specific adaptation among adult somata* (see also, Partridge and Gems 2006). Rose (2008) has argued, therefore, the most effective way to postpone ageing is via SENSE (Strategies for Engineering Negligible Senescence Evolutionarily).

In summary, both SENS and SENSE projects propose to use technological interventions to manipulate the ageing process, but the target for intervention in the SENS proposal is to repair cumulative damage via rejuvenation strategies, whereas with SENSE the goal is to manipulate the forces of natural selection such that fruit flies—and by extension, mammals—can be experimentally evolved to slow ageing and have greater life spans, and that these postponed ageing mammals could be used to reverse-engineer a slowing of human ageing. Both have the same goals—to postpone ageing (to end ageing), but the mechanism for intervention is vastly different. Nevertheless, both SENS and SENSE projects (via their main proponents Aubrey de Grey and Michael R. Rose respectively) both share a frustration, a disdain, as it were, for the incompleteness that is associated with both domains of mainstream of gerontology and geriatrics in the context of using scientific and technological means to directly address and change the course of senescence. Both de Grey and Rose accuse the establishment—the mainstream scientists in the field of ageing—of protecting their disciplinary "turf" and following rigid theoretical and methodological constraints, hamstringing any progress in postponing ageing, or ending it completely. In this regard, Rose (2008) actually gives de Grey and the SENS project credit for taking on the passivity (which corresponds to judgment that the mere compression of morbidity is lacking as an adequate and satisfactory goal for scientists in the field of ageing) in mainstream biogerontology,

> The SENS proposal has several excellent features for the mobilization of resources to conquer ageing. Most importantly, it is based on the idea that we do need to understand every particular of ageing in order to make significant medical progress. This is a very important step; otherwise the scientific field of ageing research will remain primarily an indefinite source of employment and funding for gerontologists, rather than a material aid to human well-being. (p. 532)

This notion of using science and technology to extend human well-being, eliminate suffering, eradicate disease, and conquer death itself raises questions of personal and professional motivations for both de Grey and Rose—and then the ironic connection back to the first inflection point that was described in this book—the philosophy of the ageing process—ageing *as a reflection*. It is here we must confront and address several philosophical and ethical concerns for both the SENS and SENSE projects, and the perspectives of Ray Kurzweil (whom we have briefly discussed earlier) and the entire scope of the "post ageing" enterprise as a desired and a necessary scientific and technological endeavor. That is, we must contemplate the moral and ethical concerns surrounding the postponement and ending of ageing, the conceptualization of "ageing" and "disease," and the prospect (and desirability) of physical immortality, despite the possibility (and it is here that we speculate, because we are not completely sure) that neither de Grey or Rose (or both) see little reason to address moral and ethical concerns—only in the sense that it would be immoral not to embrace scientific and technological advancements as the solution to morbidity and mortality. Both de Grey and Rose (and Kurzweil for that matter) appear to be genuinely dedicated to the cause of reducing human suffering and using their professional efforts to facilitate the enhancement of the human experience, but we detect that there is something deeper—a common thread—for both the SENSE and SENS projects that is at the intersection of historical, philosophical, theological, ethical, and metaphysical crosscurrents.

7.2 Philosophical, Theological, Ethical, and Metaphysical Concerns

The radical version of the "post ageing" inflection point (and its exemplars) is simply not satisfied with scientific advancements to merely compress morbidity, know about the causes of the how and why of ageing, optimize ageing, or to manipulate and modify only the external environments that surround the ageing individual (e.g., assistive technology)—no, the goals are more monumental with dramatic consequences for just about every sphere of human existence. In our opinion, at the very core of the motivation and operations of SENS, and SENSE, and the possibility of a technological singularity (see Goertzel 2007; Kurzweil 2005) is to move beyond ageing so that the *modus operandi* in the radical version is to modify, rejuvenate, and transcend (see Harris 2010). The goal is not to simply make the best of what we have, rather it is to make more—and better—than what we have (Garreau 2005). The radical version of post ageing will only be satisfied when scientific advancements and the use of technologies can fully intervene with the internal environment of the human body and address the ultimate "limits" of human finitude and uniqueness (the epitome of intelligence). Indeed, it is the specter of *mortality*, the presence of death as a natural outcome of human existence that is to be reckoned with assertively, and most decisively through SENS, SENSE, and Singularity.

Prior to the post ageing era, humans had the significance of a life as defined by how ageing and death were to be confronted, dealt with, and assimilated as much as possible through metaphysical and theological traditions. One was taught to overcome the fear of death (as death was inevitable and mysterious) via Stoic and Platonic exercises in thinking and rationalizations, or through the great monotheistic traditions of faith and prayer that would deliver the humble and mortal servant to immortality after death, or through the Buddhist discipline of detachment in which the past and future simply are, but are less important than the present. These approaches, these metaphysical and theological answers to the significance of ageing and the inevitability of death, are reminiscent of the previous inflection points in the study of the human life course. They are perhaps even necessary to the fabric of ageing as a *reflection*, ageing as a *problem*, ageing as a *challenge*, and even to ageing as a *reward*.

But in the post ageing domain and in this developing era of the radical version, ageing will become an *artifact*—and death will be conquered not by reasoning through and past "it" into some Gnostic and cosmic order or through a resurrection of the body and soul after death but by the destruction of the real and metaphysical wall that limits human existence and comprehension, *transcending* the assumed maximum lifespan for *Homo sapiens*. The radical version of post ageing offers the potential of immortality in the near future, perhaps within our life time, and, most importantly, *before* the specter of death can occur as something inevitable and permanent (see Seidel 2008). This new perspective within the radical version of post ageing is reflected in the statement, "Death is not a metaphysical problem anymore. It is a scientific problem, and it should be solved as soon as possible" (Goertzel 2010). This perspective has given rise to the term "death hacking" (or "bio-hacking") (Carr 2010) which describes the tinkering and beyond the edge manipulation involved in prolongevity activities, especially the ones that alter genetic material or involve technological developments in the human-machine interface. And if for most of us, this kind of transcendence (to transform beyond ageing—and death) seems beyond the human comprehension and capability, Goertzel (2010) has suggested that although the roadmap to radical human healthspan extension is clearer than ever, the biggest challenge to overcoming the "problem" of "death due to ageing" is the limitation of human thinking; that is, the effectiveness of the brains of human researchers to ask the right questions and to discover the most effective interventions. But what is the solution to this problem? Goertzel (2010) is proposing that the ultimate solution to solving the riddle of ageing and death—and thereby increasing human healthspan—and achieving Methuselarity—is with the technology; more specifically, via artificial general intelligence. In other words, an "artificial biologist" that would have the ability to think (or compute) far beyond the human brain's capability is theoretically able to solve the "limited lifespan problem."

This is very much the "heaven" scenario that Garreau (2005) discussed in his book, *Radical Evolution*, and this perspective also serves as conceptual and applied "bridge" to the potential for the *transcendence* of human nature. Thus, the movement known as transhumanism (Seidel 2008, uses the term "posthumanity") shares many, but not all, of the goals and philosophical attributes of the radical version of post ageing.

Transhumanism is a multi-layered, shape-shifting concept that embraces a vast array of descriptor terms and advocates such as: artificial intelligence, nanotechnologies, immortality, robotics, science fiction, cybernetics, futurology, postbiology, singularity, methuselarity, posthumanism, Ray Kurzweil, Aubrey de Grey and Ben Goertzel. Agar (2007) in a review of the literature on the subject, noted that transhumanism is (according to its proselytizers),

> ...the intellectual and cultural movement that affirms the possibility and desirability of fundamentally improving the human condition through applied reason, especially by developing and making widely available technologies to eliminate ageing and to greatly enhance human intellectual, physical, and psychological capacities. (p. 12)

Garreau (2005) noted that transhumanism started in the 1970s but gained more momentum as,

> ...the genetic, robotic, information and nano technologies—the GRIN technologies—make the transhumanists' interest in engineered evolution increasingly credible....Transhumanists are keen on the enhancement of human intellectual, physical and emotional capabilities, the elimination disease and unnecessary suffering, and the dramatic extension of life span. (p. 231)

However, not everyone sees the goals and activities of transhumanism as resulting in a "heaven" scenario (see also Verdoux 2009). For example, Francis Fukuyama, the author of *Our Posthuman Future*, believes that biotechnology will lead to a "hell" scenario instead (Garreau 2005). Agar (2007) indicated that Fukuyama, and others in his camp (e.g., Leon Kass, Jeremy Rifkin) are referred to (by the transhumanists) as "bioconservatives" who believe that bioengineering technologies are "distinctively threatening to our humanity" (p. 12). The distinctions between a transhumanist and bioconservative give the impression of a simple dichotomy of perspectives and attitudes and values. But this is not so. It is important for those who have an interest in gerontology issues in higher education and technology to grasp the complexity and array of perspectives better understood within a matrix of bio-political dimensions. For example, the Institute for Ethics and Emerging Technologies (IEET) has proposed several categories within the matrix: Libertarian Transhumanists, Technoprogressives, Left-wing Bioconservatives, and Right-wing Bioconservatives based on several key indicators such as definition, exemplary groups, citizenship, humanism versus religious right, individual liberty versus yuck factor, technological risks, the equality challenge of enhancement technology, procreative liberty, ecological protection, structural unemployment, and globalization. According to the information gathered from their web site (www.ieet.org), the IEET represents a technoprogressive perspective and claims to be,

> …a center for voices arguing for a responsible, constructive, ethical approach to the most powerful emerging technologies. We believe that technological progress can be a catalyst for positive human development so long as we ensure that technologies are safe and equitably distributed. We call this a "technoprogressive" orientation. We aim to showcase technoprogressive ideas about how technological progress can increase freedom, happiness, and human flourishing in democratic societies. Focusing on emerging technologies that have the potential to positively transform social conditions and the quality of human lives—especially "human enhancement technologies"—the IEET seeks to cultivate academic, professional, and popular understanding of their implications, both positive and negative, and to encourage responsible public policies for their safe and equitable use.

Although IEET prefers the label technoprogressive to transhumanist, some scholars prefer to group the entire matrix into "strong conceptions" and "moderate conceptions" of transhumanism and argue that one particular criticism, *moral arbitrariness*, undermines both forms of transhumanism (McNamee and Edwards 2009). Advocates for "strong" transhumanism are engaged in a project (with technology as the intervention) to overcome the limits (including intelligence and the human life span) of human nature, whereas the moderate project seeks to *enhance* human characteristics by augmenting it with technology (i.e., greater resistance to disease) but does not go as far as fundamentally changing human nature (McNamee and Edwards 2009). Perhaps to readers of this book the difference between overcoming and enhancing human nature might be subtle, but we like to think that moderate transhumanism has significant overlap with the moderate [5.1–5.4] version of post ageing and strong transhumanism with the radical version [5.5 and >] of post ageing. McNamee and Edwards (2009) offered a compelling "slippery slope" critique to the arbitrariness of the vague "goals" of transhumanism which appear to lack explicit specified ends as well as a failure to specify their *telos,* especially when compared to the uses of technology in the field of medicine which McNamee and Edwards claim, "…are clearly medically defined and the means regulated closely" (p. 518). In effect, McNamee and Edwards (2009) were looking for a more judicious perspective on the technologically driven agenda of transhumanism that would rise above sloganeering and emotionally laden exhortations. It was previously mentioned that the IEET identified itself as *technoprogressive*, and yet when it comes to issues related to ageing and disease, there are several editorials and submitted blog postings that reflect more of a "strong" transhumanism (or *radical* version of post ageing) as exemplified by this perspective of Colin Farrelly (2009) titled, "21st Century Humanism" (see also Farrelly 2008). We have added emphasis in the excerpts by Farrelly (2009) to indicate the key connections between ageing and transhumanism below:

> My humanist sentiments also open my eyes to the shortcomings of evolution (evident by the prevalence of chronic disease in late life) and the prevalence of *"ageism"*. If humanists reflected critically and consistently upon their basic moral convictions, I believe they would become strong advocates of *ageing research* and the aspiration to *decelerate human ageing*.
>
> A 21st century humanist recognizes the fact that no person, regardless of race, gender, nationality or *age*, deserves to suffer morbidity and mortality... For the first time in human history, most disease and death this century will occur in *late life*. *Ageing* will cause hundreds of millions of cancer deaths, strokes, bone fractures, infections, etc.
> 21st humanists ought to be among the strongest and loudest advocates of *biogerontology*... The goal of "healthy ageing" is one that follows from the core humanist sentiment that the worth of all human life, regardless of chronological age, is equal.

Based on the sentiments in the statements above, transhumanism has embraced *ageing* both as a moral imperative and as a high priority for researchers and policy-makers in alleviating suffering and disease. Furthermore, ageing issues (in the context of transhumanism) are a barometer for a new ethical standard to demonstrate actual equality and justice *across all ages* by promoting healthy ageing, presumably via enhancements and interventions using technology (see also Barclay 2009). In fact, Farrelly (2009) argues that to not *actively decelerate* the ageing process could constitute a form of ageism. Highly relevant is the fact that Farrelly (2009) credits a publication by de Grey (2005), "Life Extension, Human Rights, and the Rational Refinement of Repugnance," as the primary inspiration for Farrelly to elaborate upon the "new" transhumanism for the 21st century—including a primary focus on the ageing process. However, Muller (2007) countered with a critique against transhumanism and focused his ethical evaluation on Aubrey de Grey's SENS bioengineering program. Muller (2007) took exception to the claim that to not cure ageing is immoral and proposed instead that Aubrey's distinction of "ageing" and "disease" has important moral implications. Yet de Grey (2008) responded in kind to these critiques by reiterating his stance "that we all have a moral duty to combat ageing" and his position as far as any moral and ethical standards in the context of "ending ageing,"

> I take the view that the inexorable loss of vitality and rise in risk of death that we call "ageing" is among—indeed, possibly foremost among—the suboptimal features of life as we currently know it. Thus, I am necessarily keen to combat ageing as much as possible as soon as possible. Since society in general does not share my fervor on this matter, and since the required technological advances will undoubtedly require very considerable investment of time and money, my efforts to hasten the defeat of ageing must perforce include not only direct, scientific, contributions to the development of that technology but also contributions to the effort to bring society around to my way of thinking, thereby causing these resources to be brought to bear. (p. 5)

The debate and dialogue on the ethics and the science continues on—and most likely will as long as Aubrey de Grey sustains his tenacious drive to "end ageing" via SENS. Despite the relentless criticism from de Grey's competitors and detractors, we have to recall what Nuland (2005) said of de Grey, "He has become more than a man; he is a movement" (p. 40). And this "movement" of anti-ageing has expanded to the domain of transhumanism, which carries its own strength and limitations as far as science and ethics are concerned. And so at this point on the curvature (in the later part of the year 2010), where do we stand within the context of ethics, philosophy, and theology with regards to the implications of a radical post ageing inflection point? While we submit that we have undoubtedly moved (both in the field of ageing, gerontology, and in our society) into the post ageing inflection point (with the remnants of the other inflections points still with us) at least in the moderate version, we believe the radical version is still *emergent*. It is beyond nascent, but the full impact of the GRIN technologies on the human condition, especially in the ethical domain, is still not fully understood. Furthermore, the domain of post ageing (at least its radical version) is still in flux with many still trying to grasp the significance of the scientific foundations of projects like de Grey's SENS and Rose's SENSE. For some, these projects may represent yet another example of "fashionable nonsense" (Sokal and Bricmont 1998). Or with Nuland's (2005) original question regarding de Grey: *Is he nuts?* In other words, is all of this motivation and passion and conviction in ending ageing, moving beyond the reasonable goals of the compression of morbidity and/or optimal ageing (towards a post ageing), just really science fiction, the delusions of well-meaning scientists with a techno-messiah complex? Some, like Bainbridge (2007) have suggested that we need to embrace the inevitable convergence of science and technologies (e.g., nanotechnology, biotechnology, information technology, and cognitive technology), which will also dramatically affect human destiny by creating a new foundation of ethical decision-making (see also Seidel 2008). Some, like DeLashmutt (2006), have argued that the goals, beliefs, attitudes, and activities of transhumanism—and by extrapolation, *post ageing*—are a posthuman vision of a post biological future,

> A common theme in the myth of posthuman speculative science is the belief that advanced forms of information technology will in the future be able to accommodate radical life extension. The ability to employ technology to stave off death as long as possible had given the posthuman speculative scientists mentioned below [Moravec, Tipler, Kurzweil] a sense of confidence in their craft's ability to bring an ultimate solution to the problem of finitude, especially when cast in terms of personal mortality. (p. 274)

This is a very perceptive analysis for the many representatives who advocate for a transhumanistic transformation in the near future. It is also a possibly valid critique for those who envision a radical version of post ageing, where human life extension is altered and manipulated with the ultimate goal of immortality—thus ending ageing and, it is assumed, disease and suffering as well. In other words, are the motivation, desire, and the obsessive drive to conquer ageing and death a reflection of a very human denial relating to the existential finality of life? Is it in fact a manifestation of that universal fear of the metaphysical unknown beyond death to which theology and adherents in the various faiths claim to have insight and answers?

We cannot know what role intrapersonal dynamics or existential fears hold in influencing the attitudes of those like Ray Kurzweil (2005), in his book, *The Singularity Is Near*, where he presents his optimistic belief in the achievement of a "human level artificial intelligence by 2029, followed by an AI-triggered radical transformation of mind, society and economy by roughly 2045" (Goertzel 2007, p. 1162). The same can be asked of Aubrey de Grey (2009) and his quest for "Methuselarity," although Nuland's (2005) article did offer some tantalizing perspectives on the deeper motivations for de Grey's work with the SENS project and his quest to "end ageing." Is de Grey's passion and advocacy for SENS and "longevity escape velocity" and "regenerative medicine" the result of a hyper-driven fear and denial of the process of ageing, disease, and decline? Or, is it rather the sincere belief, a deeply held one, that technology can deliver us from morbidity and mortality, and that through manipulation of biotechnologies in particular, we will essentially live forever? Or is it that de Grey simply wants to be "unreasonable" with the status quo of mainstream biogerontology and take on the establishment to finally move beyond the traditional pattern of discovering and rather, doing something about it? This sounds very much like the old saying, "Everybody talks about the weather, but nobody does anything about it." The "it" in this case is, of course, ageing. Some may see de Grey as the ultimate pseudoscientific *Don Quixote,* a charlatan tilting at windmills, at best a "troll" that has become too enamored of the potential in technology and the possibility for complete human rejuvenation to defeat not only morbidity but mortality as well. Pontin (2006) wrote in *Technology Review* that de Grey has fallen into the role of "technological messiah" and Pontin countered the radical version of post ageing with a more limited perspective of technology in the future,

> When technology appropriates the transcendental, it becomes science fiction. Transcendence is not a part of this world, or any world that we know directly. We are alone with ourselves, and even if the application of biotechnology to human nature made us something else, we would remain creatures limited in space, time, and knowledge. Technology is most useful when it is most human in scope. Then, technology offers something close to happiness (even if ultimate happiness eludes us) by providing us with more expansive lives.

But that perspective drew criticism and led to the *Technology Review's* $20,000 challenge (see Pontin 2006) to disprove Aubrey de Grey's anti-ageing proposals. As you recall, the judges determined that none of the proposals adequately disproved the SENS project. Nevertheless, Pontin (2006) offered his own interpretation of the debate process and its results,

> In short, SENS is highly speculative. Many of its proposals have not been reproduced, nor could they be reproduced with today's scientific knowledge and technology. Echoing Myhrvold, we might charitably say that de Grey's proposals exist in a kind of antechamber of science, where they wait (possibly in vain) for independent verification. SENS does not compel the assent of many knowledgeable scientists; but neither is it demonstrably wrong.

Yet many people see in de Grey a maverick technologist with the courage and intelligence to act with fervor and dedication in conquering ageing, and as leader and exemplar in guiding—and challenging us—toward the goal of post ageing.

But as Garreau (2005) has aptly described in his book, *Radical Evolution*, the means to achieve the goal of post ageing—via the GRIN technologies—may not lead us to a "heaven" scenario. Other possible outcomes of the rapid expansion of technological developments are the "hell" scenario—that could lead to the destruction of our species, or the "prevail" scenario—the middle path where humans muddle through incrementally, keeping a tight rein on technological advancements (Garreau 2005).

Regardless of which path one believes we are on, there is the clear recognition and acknowledgement that technology has already made a dramatic impact on the human condition across the life course. The intersection of technology and ageing issues is substantial and significant and we propose that we have entered into a new inflection point beyond, and different than, the prevailing viewpoint of optimal ageing [4.0] and this inflection point has rapidly transformed from a *moderate* version and into a *radical* version. The previous goals of compression of morbidity and optimizing ageing are in danger of being swept aside by a new goal: to end ageing by enhancing and rejuvenating the human body with the surfacing tools and techniques (associated with the GRIN technologies). But not everyone is convinced that ending ageing and seeking immortality is even ethically responsible, or economically or ecologically feasible. And yet, the potential for the radical evolution of enhancing bodies and minds is now present and will continue to amplify and accelerate in the near future (Garreau 2005).

For some, technology is the solution, the answer, and the salvation. Senescence is the dis-ease to be eradicated; the second half of life is to be the time for rejuvenation; and death is to be relegated as a remnant of the past, a time when humans were limited by biological clocks and built massive theological and philosophical structures to house the mortal coil that viewed life as something finite and existentially tentative—*memento mori*. For others, technology is the enhancement, the servant, the path to the optimization of the ageing experience. And for yet others, the use of technology in engineering human life beyond the natural life span is viewed as narcissistic, escapist, and the ultimate expression of human denial, the mechanism to assume the role of both god and devil. I find it fascinating that the story of Goethe's *Faust* resonates with the theme of seeking eternal youth and ultimate knowledge, and the mechanism to achieve both is through the manipulation of the organic body with magic potions—a witch's brew. Here is an exchange between Mephistopheles and Faust (brought to our attention with an article by Berry 2009, p. 16) where the witches concoct a brew to make Faust young again. Faust can barely stomach the potion, and so he wonders if there is another way to reverse the ageing process,

Faust:
Has neither Nature nor some noble mind
Discovered some remedy, some balsam?

Mephistopheles:
There is a natural way to make you young...
Go out in a field
And start right to work, dig, hoe,
Keep your thoughts and yourself in that field,
Eat the food you raise...
Be willing to manure the field your harvest.
And that's the best way—take it from me!
To go on being young at eighty.

But Faust is not happy with that prospect either. In fact, it sounds like a passage from Virgil's *Georgics* or Voltaire's prescription for life, "Cultivate your garden." In other words, "work hard all your life and hope for the best". Bring forward that message of Goethe's *Faust* into our contemporary interest in post ageing where there is very much the theme of the manipulation of the body (via biotechnologies) as a "natural" way to make us young again, and forever. But there is also the specter of what technology represents in terms of breaking away from the "old" in order to create something completely new, without any trappings to the past. The classical story of *Faust* should give us pause to contemplate what Faustian bargains are in store for us when we embrace technologies that could alter the human life span, change the rules and the measurement when gauging the purpose and meaning to life itself. What are we chasing in all of this technological activity? Is it the sense that we can finally break free from the old world that is morbidity and mortality and create a new world, free from the tyranny of senescence?

We propose that we as professionals should take heed to these technological developments that are rapidly altering the landscape of understanding both the *how* and the *why* of ageing—and more dramatically, quickly forcing the controversial topic upon all of us—*why age at all?* In other words, if we find the prospect of eternal youth and immortality as the desired goal, if we can finally rid ourselves of disease and pain and suffering associated with senescence, and if we transcend the biological destiny of our species into some posthuman/post biological entity, then what was ageing ever good for? What were the purpose, the function, and the essence of living into the second half of life? Is ageing meaning-*ful* or meaning-*less*? Can the ageing process be any part of what Luc Ferry (2005) refers to as "the good life", especially in the context of a 21st century technological world that may come to see "ageing" as the *problem* to be repaired and rejuvenated (see Derkx 2009; Vincent 2006). This leads to the final section of this book where we will summarize the issues linked with the evolution of inflection points in gerontology and briefly discuss the implications of the post ageing inflection point for educators who teach about the subject of ageing and those who have an interest in the philosophical issues of post-ageing.

References

Agar, N. (2007). Where to transhumanism? The literature reaches a critical mass. *Hastings Center Report, 37*(3), 12–17.

Bainbridge, W. S. (2007). Converging technologies and human destiny. *Journal of Medicine and Philosophy, 32*, 197–216.

Barclay, L. (2009). Egalitarianism and responsibility in the genetic future. *Journal of Medicine and Philosophy, 34*, 119–134.

Berry, W. (2009, December). The necessity of agriculture. *Harper's Magazine*, 15-16.

Bourke, A. F. G. (2007). Kin selection and the evolutionary theory of ageing. *Annual Review of Ecology Evolution and Systematics, 38*, 103–128.

Carr, P. (2010). Sorry deathhackers: Life is short, and so it should be. *TechCrunch*. Retrieved August 1, 2010, from http://techcrunch.com/2010/08/01/what-kills-us-makes-us-stronger.

Critser, G. (2010). *Eternity soup: Inside the quest to end ageing*. New York: Harmony Books.

de Grey, A. D. N. J. (2005). Life extension, human rights, and the rational refinement of repugnance. *Journal of Medical Ethics, 31*, 659–663.

de Grey, A. D. N. J. (2008). Is the quest to defeat ageing ethical? In S. Wint (Ed.), *Ethical futures*. Retrieved from http://sensf.com/files/sens/RSA-PP.pdf.

de Grey, A. D. N. J. (2009). The singularity and the methuselarity: Similarities and differences. *Studies in Health Technology and Informatics, 149*, 195–202.

DeLashmutt, M. W. (2006). A better life through information technology? The techno-theological eschatology of posthuman speculative science (Perspectives on techno-science and human nature). *Zygon, 41*, 267–287.

Derkx, P. (2009). Engineering substantially prolonged human life spans: Biotechnological enhancement and ethics. In R. Edmondson & H. Kondratowitz (Eds.), *Valuing older people: A humanist approach to ageing* (pp. 177–198). Bristol: The Policy Press.

Farrelly, C. (2008). Ageing research: Priorities and aggregation. *Public Health Ethics, 1*, 258–267.

Farrelly, C. (2009). 21st century humanism. *The new enlightenment*. Retrieved October 29, 2009, from http://colinfarrelly.blogspot.com/2009/10/21st-century-humanism.html.

Ferry, L. (2005). *The good life*. Chicago: University of Chicago Press.

Garreau, J. (2005). *Radical evolution: the promise and peril of enhancing our minds, our bodies—and what it means to be human*. New York: Broadway (Random House).

Goertzel, B. (2007). Human-level artificial intelligence and the possibility of a technological singularity—A reaction to Ray Kurzweil's the singularity is near, and McDermott's critique of Kurzweil. *Artificial Intelligence, 171*, 1161–1173.

Goertzel, B. (2010). *AI against ageing—AIs, superflies, and the path to immortality*. Paper presented at the Singularity Summit, August 14–15, 2010. Hyatt Regency, San Francisco, CA: Retrieved from http://www.singularitysummit.com/abstracts/goertzel.

Goldsmith, T. C. (2008). Ageing, evolvability, and the individual benefit requirement; medical implications of ageing theory controversies. *Journal of Theoretical Biology, 252*, 764–768.

Hamilton, W. D. (1966). The moulding of senescence by natural selection. *Journal of Theoretical Biology, 12*, 12–45.

Harris, J. (2010). Human enhancement. *The Philosophers' Magazine*, 50 (Third Quarter), 62–63.

Hawkes, K., O'Connell, J. F., Blurton Jones, N. G., Alvarez, H., & Charnov, E. L. (1998). Grandmothering, menopause, and the evolution of human life histories. *PNAS, 95*(3), 1336–1339.

Kurzweil, R. (2005). *The singularity is near: When humans transcend biology*. New York: Penguin Books.

Lithgow, G. J. (2006). Why ageing isn't regulated: A lamentation on the use of language in ageing literature. *Experimental Gerontology, 41*, 890–893.

Ljubuncic, P., & Reznick, A. (2009). The evolutionary theories of ageing revisited—A mini-review. *Gerontology, 55*, 205–216.

McNamee, M. J., & Edwards, S. D. (2009). Transhumanism, medical technology, and slippery slopes. *Journal of Medical Ethics, 32*, 513–518.

Martin, G. (2005). How is the evolutionary theory of ageing holding up against mounting attacks? *American Ageing Association Newsletter*, April, 6–8.

Martin, G. (2006). Keynote lecture: An update on the what, why, and how questions of ageing. *Experimental Gerontology, 41*, 460–463.
Mittledorf, J., & Pepper, J. (2009). Senescence as an adaption to limit the spread of disease. *Journal of Theoretical Biology*, (Sept.), 186–195.
Muller, F. S. (2007). On futuristic gerontology: A philosophical evaluation of Aubrey de Grey's SENS Project. *International Journal of Applied Philosophy, 21*(2), 225–239.
Nuland, J. (2005). Do you want to live forever? *MIT Technology Review*. Retrieved from http://www.technologyreview.com/featuredstory/403654/do-you-want-to-live-forever/.
Partridge, L., & Gems, D. (2006). Beyond the evolutionary theory of ageing, from functional genomics to evo-gero. *Trends in Ecology & Evolution, 21*, 334–340.
Pontin, J. (2006). Is defeating ageing only a dream? *Technology Review*. Retrieved from http://www.technologyreview.com/sens/.
Rose, M. R. (2005). *The long tomorrow: How advances in evolutionary biology can help us postpone ageing*. New York: Oxford University Press.
Rose, M. R. (2008). Making SENSE: Strategies for engineering negligible senescence evolutionarily. *Rejuvenation Research, 11*(2), 527–534.
Rose, M. R. (2009). Adaptation, ageing, and genomic information. *Ageing, 1*(5), 444–450.
Rose, M. R., Rauser, C. L., Benford, G., Matos, M., & Mueller, L. D. (2007). Hamilton's forces of natural selection after forty years. *Evolution, 61*(6), 1265–1276.
Seidel, A. (2008). *Inhuman thoughts: Philosophical explorations of posthumanity*. Lanham: Lexington Books.
Sell, C., Lorenzini, A., & Brown-Borg, H. (Eds.). (2009). *Life-span extension: Single-cell organisms to man*. New York: Humana Press.
Sokal, A., & Bricmont, J. (1998). *Fashionable nonsense: Postmodern intellectuals' abuse of science*. New York: Picador.
Stipp, D. (2010). *The youth pill: Scientists at the brink of an anti-ageing revolution*. New York: Current (Penguin).
Verdoux, P. (2009). Transhumanism, progress and future. *Journal of Evolution and Technology, 20*(2), 49–69.
Vincent, J. (2006). Ageing contested: Anti-ageing science and the cultural construction of old age. *Sociology, 40*(4), 681–698.
Weiner, J. (2010). *Long for this world: The strange science of immortality*. New York: HarperCollins.

Part III
The Next Inflection Point

Chapter 8
The Promise and Challenges of Post Ageing

Abstract We are not convinced that the inflection point of *optimal ageing* is the ultimate culmination and apogee of all that we have done—and will do—in the domain of gerontology and geriatrics. We are most certain that a burgeoning inflection point has arrived and made an impact by challenging our received views within the "ageing enterprise." We submit that the GRIN technologies will disrupt and flip on its head each and every previous inflection point and its attendant prevailing view. In the past, *ageing* has been the optic by which we reflect on decline and mortality, problem-solve the symptoms of senescence, enact policies to buffer the demographic transitions, and promote lifestyles, attitudes, diets, and outlooks that will reframe the later years into civic engagement, wisdom, and legacy. But that was then, and this is now, when we will have to make room for this new perspective of "post ageing", even the radical versions, in our classrooms, conferences, and publications. Despite the heated rhetoric and polemics that have been associated with "anti-ageing medicine" and human life extension, the intersection of technology and ageing is substantial and significant.

Keywords Ageing philosophy · Gerontologists · Geriatricians · Methuselarity · Singularity · Transhumanism

We began this book by examining the historical development of gerontology as a field of study, a taxonomy, an approach, a lexicon. As an industry and a profession, gerontology has a checkered and dendritic course of progression, and while many have attempted to profile the major events and the prevailing streams of philosophy and thought along the way, we have proposed an alternative perspective that offers an "inflection point" heuristic. Our viewpoint avoids the epistemological trappings of the term "paradigm", especially as it relates to the interdisciplinary field of ageing. We proposed that there have been five major inflection points in the extant history of gerontological scholarship and practice:

K.F. Felsted and S.D. Wright, *Toward Post Ageing*,
Healthy Ageing and Longevity 1, DOI 10.1007/978-3-319-09051-1_8

Inflection Points (Directional Shifts in Prevailing Theme in Gerontology/Ageing)
[1.0]: Philosophy of Ageing (ageing as a *reflection*)
[2.0]: Bio-medical Diseases of Ageing (ageing as a *problem*)
[3.0]: Demographics of Ageing (ageing as a *challenge*)
[4.0]: Optimal Ageing (ageing as a *reward*)
5.0: Post Ageing (ageing as an *artifact*)

We further proposed that the optimal ageing theme has been the predominant pathway and compass within the gerontological literature for at least the last two decades but that a new direction, driven by bioengineering and technology, has already surfaced in our contemporary era. We reviewed both the moderate and radical versions of the [5.0] post ageing inflection point, based on the typology of Garreau's (2005) GRIN technologies. We also indicated that the radical version does not simply represent an overturning or replacement of the scientific management of ageing, but rather has metamorphosed into a "scientific-technological" *Weltanschauung* that seeks to move beyond ageing (into post ageing) as a necessary phase in the life course. In other words, ageing (biologically, socially, and psychologically) is something to be overcome and transcended—first incrementally and then completely. The *radical* version of post ageing has monumental implications for the domains of both gerontology and geriatrics. Many of us who teach, conduct research, and provide service in the field of ageing have probably been operating under the traditional banner of scientific management of ageing, within a humanities framework, or both, and may find the goals of post ageing in the radical version to be untenable, extreme, pseudo-scientific, unethical and without moral foundation. Some will even view these goals as wholly characteristic of ageist tendencies that deny the reality of both the ageing process as a natural consequence of human development and mortality as the inevitable consequence of being alive (see Vincent 2006).

Our traditional training and pedagogical focus is on scanning the literature and databases for gathering and weaving the "usual suspects" of conceptual models and theoretical structures into the classroom setting for students to learn and hopefully "buy into." And as we have stated before, we can be hard pressed to even find relevant and informative examples in that regard. Bench scientists stay focused on the *how* and *why* of ageing and reveal the latest discoveries on the *causes* of ageing. Our clinical practice seeks to treat the burdens of frailty with medical treatments and to alleviate the pain and suffering accompanying chronic conditions and uses the compression of morbidity as a paradigmatic guiding light. As practitioners in the field, we target assistance to those who seek to age-in-place and highlight the latest cost-saving strategies in the ageing industry. Tenured researchers seek extramural funding and drill down into the multi-layered datasets, plan for the challenges of demographic transitions with impressive statistical models, or gather empirical findings that suggest ways extend the health and wellness of the individual into the supercentenarian years. Yet, as gerontologists and geriatricians and professionals in allied fields, we rarely entertain the notion, discuss the significance, understand the process, or debate the implications of technological interventions to repair, rejuvenate, regenerate, and enhance the human body and mind as a way *to end ageing*. This is understandable, given the engrained view that our careers, business, and *raison d'être* are to discover, understand, and treat what is supposed to be the *given*: "it" (ageing) is axiomatic, and not optional. We assume ageing to be something as fundamental to the experience of life as thinking and breathing are.

While we can wrap layers of reflection and philosophical nostrums around it, or see it as a problem that propels us to work diligently "maximiz[ing] functional independence and quality of life during the years of frailty" (Fillit and Butler 2009, p. 351), or elevate the enormity of demographic transitions (i.e., the baby boomers) that they form the tsunami that is either economically threatening or culture transforming, or we acknowledge the *fact* of ageing but then gloss the experience with "successful ageing" or "healthy ageing" or "optimal ageing" strategies to make the most out of life—we will still drop in front of the wall of mortality at our maximum life span. In any case, the dividend of the longevity revolution is to promote and experience optimal ageing.

But we are not convinced that the inflection point of *optimal ageing* is the ultimate culmination and apogee of all that we have done—and will do—in the domain of gerontology and geriatrics. We are most certain that a burgeoning inflection point has arrived and made an impact by challenging our received views within the "ageing enterprise." We submit that the GRIN technologies will disrupt and flip on its head each and every previous inflection point and its attendant prevailing view. In the past, *ageing* has been the optic by which we reflect on decline and mortality, problem-solve the symptoms of senescence, enact policies to buffer the demographic transitions, and promote lifestyles, attitudes, diets, and outlooks that will reframe the later years into civic engagement, wisdom, and legacy. But that was then, and this is now, when we will have to make room for this new perspective of "post ageing", even the radical versions, in our classrooms, conferences, and publications. Despite the heated rhetoric and polemics that have been associated with "anti-ageing medicine" and human life extension, the intersection of technology and ageing is substantial and significant.

In a larger context, technology (techne) has already transformed the economy (Brynjolfsson and Saunders 2010); the arts (Plate and Smelik 2009; Reichle 2009); patterns of history (Barzun 2000); human intelligence (Hawkins 2004); literature and architecture (Brodsky 2009); engineering on the nanoscale (Jones 2004); medicine on the nanoscale (Schulz et al. 2009); our perceptions of human nature (Garreau 2005) and spirituality (via Kevin Kelly) (see Lawler 2010); the way we forget, recall, and remember (Bell and Gemmell 2009; Katz and Peters 2008; Mayer-Schonberger 2009); the way we think or don't think (Bauerlein 2008; Bowman 2008; Carr 2008; Cascio 2009; Cooper 2009);the way we express love (Pettman 2006); and the way we connect—and should not connect (Powers 2010). Technology has already been employed as a way to extend the cognitive circuitry of individual minds (Clark 2007, 2010), as a technique to serve as replacement parts (neural prostheses) for the brain (Berger and Glanzman 2005), and as a way to restore functional tissue in humans (Atala et al. 2010), and all of this will force the re-examination of the core issues of what makes us human (e.g., freedom, love, will, control, destiny). But the various intersections of technology with humanity are never embraced with unconditional acceptance. Arthur (2009) is his book, *The Nature of Technology—What It Is and How Evolves*, succinctly captures the tension between technology as serving our live sand directing our lives,

> If we merely used nature's phenomena in raw form, to power water wheels or propel sailing ships, we would feel more at home with technology, and our trust and hope would be less at odds. But now, with the coming of genetic engineering, machine intelligence, bionics, climate engineering, we are beginning to use technology—use nature—to intervene directly within nature...We fear this phenomena of technology that is not in our control. We fear we are unleashing something of disembodied action somehow taking on a life of its own and coming somehow to control us. We fear technology as a living thing that will bring us death. Not fear of death of nothingness, but a worse death. The death that comes with no-freedom. The death of will. (p. 215)

And perhaps this is a major factor in the ambivalence in considering a *full* post ageing inflection point for gerontology and geriatrics. On one hand, the moderate version of post ageing appears to be serving our lives as ageing individuals with assistive technologies to better our life experiences and to optimize our well-being further and further along the life course until the last remaining months of life, which is what we associate with maximum life span (hopefully, disability-free). But to also consider the opportunity to extend human life beyond the natural life span by using technologies associated with the radical version of post ageing raises a host of concerns (and fears) that crosscut ethics, morality, economics, and environmental issues. One of these is the fear that some technologies will escape human design and control and end up as either wrecking havoc to the environment or becoming malevolent entities seeking to destroy the humanity that created it. Thus we need to recognize that developing technologies will not only permeate in both breadth and depth the structure of how we envision ourselves as ageing entities but also how we judge and evaluate ageing as something to be understood—as well as something to be dramatically altered, manipulated, eradicated, and perhaps, become an *artifact* of our own doing. Although we believe it is important to address the moderate and radical versions of post ageing using Socratic "lessons" (see Eisele 2009) in the classroom setting with our students, we do not believe it is necessarily our role as gerontology professionals to advocate that the radical version is the de facto path we wish to take as a society. But we will all need to be engaged in this discussion and we need to begin as soon as possible (see Partridge et al. 2009). As scientists and educators we need to appreciate the full spectrum of arguments for and against the use of GRIN technologies in relation to enhancing the body and mind and understand how both rational thinking and emotional responses are a part of the human discourse on a highly charged topic in science (see Macilwain 2009; Specter 2009).

But awareness and discussion of the GRIN technologies among both teachers and students in the field of ageing is only one dimension of a post ageing inflection point; another dimension will have to be the return to the philosophical dimension of ageing [1.0] which centers on the discourse of the humanities (see Gay 2010; Rickman 2004), and the contemplation of life in the context of finite time and space (or the antithesis thereof), the purpose and meaning of life as situated in mortality (or the antithesis thereof) (see Cole et al. 2010), and the examination of what constitutes the "good life" in the presence of senescence (or the antithesis thereof). In other words, we must as the current custodians and stewards of an interdisciplinary approach to the study of ageing consider the ramifications and consequences, the prospects and prognostications, the strengths and limitations, and the substance and significance for any post ageing experience now—and for all of those who would follow in generations to come. Ironically, one of the positive consequences of the emergence of the post ageing inflection point is the parallel renaissance of a deeper rumination about the ageing process and the significance of senescence in the life course. We have in fact entered into what Kaufman (2010) has referred to as the "age of reflexive longevity" which captures the essence of dialogue and debate about what is "natural ageing" and "normal ageing" and "disease" and "pathology." Kaufman noted that,

> Most recently, developments in the bioscience have encouraged the view that ageing is a treatable disease. Rapidly expanding knowledge of the human genome, together with advances in tissue engineering, the bioengineering of drugs, and the ability to manipulate cellular ageing genetically, creates social expectations about applications of genetic technologies to cure the diseases of later life, stave off death, and alter the "natural" process of ageing. These goals have become intertwined and largely inseparable (p. 229).

We submit that since these issues associated with post ageing are so intertwined and inseparable, what is needed is a rejuvenation and re-emphasis of the first inflection point—the philosophical—(ageing as "reflection") that would serve not as counterweight, but as a complementary and concomitant activity in the post ageing era.

8.1 The Intersection of Inflection Points: [1.0] Philosophy (Ageing as a *Reflection*) and [5.0] Post Ageing (Ageing as an *Artifact*)

> When philosophy paints its grey in grey, one form of life has become old, and by means of grey, it cannot be rejuvenated, but only known. The owl of Minerva takes it flight only, when the shades of night are gathering.
>
> Author's Preface, *Philosophy of Right*
>
> Georg H.W. Hegel 1820
> (translation S.W. Dyde, March 23, 1896)

> Philosophy is indeed concerned with reality, but not to discover new facts about it: it seeks to improve our understanding of what we already know. It does not seek to observe more, but to clarify our vision of what we see.
>
> The Nature and Future of Philosophy
> Michael Dummett (2010)

Some may wonder why we advocate for the return of philosophical concepts and methods (see Baggini and Fosl 2010) to the field of ageing [1.0], and why we think the re-tooling is critically needed as we proceed into the post ageing inflection point [5.0]. Indeed, on the surface it appears that the two inflection points have little in common with one inflection point (philosophy) appearing to be quite antiquated and associated with a "pre-scientific" mode of thinking, while the other one (post ageing) appears to be quite futuristic and fast moving. In fact, it appears that one inflection point assumes the ageing process as an ontological given [1.0] while the other [5.x] seeks to demolish the process such that the experience of ageing has the potential to be completely negated. Waxing philosophical about ageing is so *yesterday*, while engaging post ageing is so—*tomorrow*. It would be a valid proposition to advance, that gerontology and philosophy have *not* enjoyed a fruitful exchange when compared to the cumulative activity that we associate with the scientific method and its approach and the field of ageing. But another key element related to the dominant focus of science in the field of ageing (vs. philosophy) has to do with perspective and purpose of each activity.

For example, when we ponder Hegel's philosophical perspective regarding the role of philosophy in the grand scheme of understanding our situation—our reality—and our existence, it appears that philosophy has less to do with teaching what the world ought to be (future possibilities), and instead, its attention and focus is on what has already happened. Philosophy appears to work best when looking in the rear view mirror, while science and technology look through the windshield. In other words, philosophy (at least from the Hegelian perspective) cannot be prescriptive because it understands only in hindsight, thus the owl of Minerva takes its flight only when the shades of night are gathering. This raises the question of what possible value is reflection and philosophical inquiry to the realm of post ageing when "it" (i.e., GRIN technologies) has already taken place and seemingly appears to be moving at near light speed (toward *Singularity*? toward *Methuselarity*?), while philosophy plods along at glacial speed and is left to ponder on the dust kicked up by the scientific/technological rocket of post ageing leaving the earth's gravitational pull. Philosophy seems destined for retrospection, while science and technology advance prospectively. To add even more irony to our proposal for the active intersection of philosophy (ageing as reflection) and post ageing (ageing as artifact) is the potential for many to consider the two inflection points to be *mutually exclusive* on two counts; (1) any discussion or debate on the topic of technology and ageing (post ageing) is (or should be) outside the realm of philosophy and is purely a "scientific/technical" debate (see Vincent 2006); and (2) if one starts with the position that human ageing is primarily a biological process capable of technical control, then the possibility of having life *not* to grow old (as we think we know it) makes the philosophical inquiry on ageing (as reflection) a moot point. There is nothing to understand or clarify: it is to age—or not to age. There is no opportunity to paint gray in gray, or to reflect on life's journey at all, because in post ageing, there may be no dusk to gather at the end of the day, or an owl to offer wisdom taking flight. Rather, the entire notion of reflection upon past events (both historical and individual developmental) is turned on its head so that Hegel's owl is transformed into a rooster that is perpetually crowing at daybreak. Such is the strange new world of post ageing where the philosophical perspectives of Sophocles (in the play *Oedipus at Colonus*), *those* of the Roman stoics (as with *Seneca*: *On the Shortness of Life*, translation by Costa 2005), and those of Marcus Aurelius, the philosopher-king, from his work *Meditations*, would seem out of joint with their collective blunt philosophical message: We are born to die, and for many the span of life is shortened considerably due to a lack of care in valuing the time that is allotted, and in the bigger picture of history and infinite time, a lifetime is enough given the trials of existence. But then again, the *measuring stick* (average life expectancy) for a life lived is vastly different for us today than it was for Sophocles, Seneca or Marcus Aurelius. In the domain of post ageing, it would appear that such philosophical perspectives are perhaps no longer viable nor relevant in the contemporary world of scientific models, postmodernism, longevity revolutions, optimal ageing, supercentenarians, and GRIN technologies, and the prospect of post ageing.

Perhaps. But maybe this *is* exactly the right time for a deeper consideration, a reconsideration, of the value and the purpose of reflection in our lives as ageing individuals. In the final section of this book, we are proposing a provocative dynamic that relates to all of the inflection points in the heuristic we have been discussing thus far, but where there is a particular—and ironically, much needed—discourse between the first and last inflection points. In other words, it is ironic that the trend in post ageing (especially with the radical version) is toward the complete emancipation of the human being from the experiential process of ageing, but at the same time, in parallel fashion, we also see the need for a substantial revisit, or better yet, a *rejuvenation* of the role for the inflection point of the *philosophy of ageing*. We are calling for a renaissance of the first inflection point that examines *ageing as a reflection. We see this* as a critical and concurrent activity in tandem with the emergent inflection point of [5.0], especially in context with the advocacy and implementation of GRIN technologies [5.5 and >] as a mechanism to *end ageing*—and as it alters the ontological status of what it means to have a life as well as the metaphysical status of what it means to have a "good life" in the age of technology (see Thagard 2010).

But again—*why?* Why are not the scientific and/or technological methods sufficient in capturing the essence of post ageing—or for that matter, any inflection point within the field of ageing? What could a philosophical vantage point offer in terms of any additional significance and substance to the prospect of post ageing? Why is there the need for the intersect? First, we must consider the different roles that science and philosophy can bring to the domain of post ageing. A good place to start would be the clarification of how science and philosophy are complementary while operating separately. Here is Dummett (2010) with a succinct overview,

> Science and philosophy are not rivals; both are concerned to improve our picture of reality, but in quite different ways. Science supplies us with ever more facts about reality, although to do so, it has often to fashion new concepts in terms of which to state those facts. It thus enlarges our field of vision. Philosophy seeks to rectify our vision, enabling us, as Wittgenstein said, to see the world aright, including those features of the world that science reveals. It does so by the slow, laborious process of clarifying our concepts, both our everyday concepts and the new concepts introduced by science. The two are complementary: both are engaged in mankind's long quest for truth (p. 30).

Further elucidations for the role of science and philosophy in the professional and university settings were provided by several contributors (Brooks 2010; Deneen 2010; Kenneally 2010); in a symposium on "Science, the Humanities, and the University" in the publication, *The New Atlantis*: *A Journal of Technology & Society*. Our goal for citing this publication is to indicate that despite the complementary role of science and philosophy, the two domains have nevertheless drifted apart, with philosophy placed in a secondary position of relevancy. For example, Kenneally (2010) reflected on the evolution of the modern American university and highlighted the tensions between philosophy and science, their different perspectives, and how Cartesian science and rational productivity has dominated the landscape of education (thus, the advancing rise of the technocratic university) at the expense of the "passive and noble contemplation" that is the "philosophic eros." Deneen (2010) noted how a new science no longer sought to *understand* the world and its creatures, but to *transform* them. Deneen (2010) went on to propose that while science has displaced the humanities, it has

> ...made modern humanity increasingly subject to a kind of ungovernable hubris. Ultimately modern science aspires to reach beyond the mastery of nature to the mastery of human nature, the last frontier for it dominion. This displacement of the humanities has led inevitably to a Gnostic disdain for the human. (p. 61)

This critique of modern science—and for that matter, modern technology—has a direct relevancy to the goals of transhumanism, the concept of singularity, and of methuselarity, and important implications for reflecting upon the trends in post ageing. That is to say, what is it exactly that post ageing hopes to accomplish? And do we grasp that transforming the human is not the same as understanding the human? For example, Brooks (2010) uses the philosophical perspectives of Nietzsche to emphasize the demarcation between science/scientists and philosophy/philosophers,

> What then can Nietzsche's discussion of scientists and philosophers teach those of us who are trying to determine the standpoint from which we ought to approach the problems and questions that confront every human being? To begin, Nietzsche teaches us that we ought to approach these problems and questions from the standpoint of precisely what we are—that is, from the standpoint of beings whose lives consist in affirming, denying, preferring, and loving—and not from the standpoint of scientific objectivity or neutrality. (p. 102)

Brooks (2010) proposes that studying philosophy actually encourages a non-objective or "unscientific" style of thinking that can counter the dehumanizing effects of excessive exposure to scientific education. In other words, a philosophical approach embraces personal opinion and subjectivity, but also forces us to review and reflect on how and why we find affinity to such perspectives.

But our goal here is not to revisit the nuances of the supposed "two cultures" debate (or even one or three cultures) (Davenport 1970; Gay 2010; Kagan 2009; Snow 1964) or to further discuss the impact and role of "scientism" in general (Sorell 1991; Stenmark 2001) or its supposed impact in the field of ageing; rather, our intent is to consider the potential for a stronger *philosophical orientation* in evaluating, understanding, and critically reviewing the role of science and technology (especially the radical version of post ageing) in the ageing experience. Thus, we are in agreement with Tauber (2009) and his perspectives in his book, *Science and the Quest for Meaning*, that there is a need to broaden the ethos of science to expand the landscape of reason in the post-positivist era,

> Further, once we understand a wider array of values as contributing to scientific knowledge and allow them their rightful place in the calculus of knowing, opportunity beckons for science to join a larger menu of concerns than its traditional twin roles of supporting technological innovation and mastery of nature (p. 14).

As the field enters into the post ageing inflection point, we propose that it is of paramount importance to philosophically examine *how and why* humanistic and trans-humanistic interests and values influence the science that drives that technology (the "industry") associated with post ageing scholarship and interventional activities. We hope for a philosophical examination of how the scientific enterprise contributes to the metaphysical orientation such that ageing and mortality are now seen as variable and optional to the lived experience—and not as a given (Small 2007). For example, Baars (2010) has suggested that Manheimer's (2000) philosophical matrix of themes for human loss and gain be expanded to include the technocratic "anti-ageing" programs,

> …that present themselves as the spearhead of fundamental scientific research but may, besides pursuing more mundane goals also be seen as contemporary representatives of old magical traditions (p. 107).

Baars (2010) went on to say that the quest to end ageing could be interpreted as a "dialectic of enlightenment" which is the desire to engage in a technically advanced control of nature and representation (and regression) to a primitive form of magic and myth (ex. the fountain of youth). Baars (2010) elaborated the thesis in this fashion,

> As long as the ageing process remains uncontrollable, the striving for complete technological control is continually confronted with mankind's shortcoming, which explains why those who are reminders of this tragic failure tend to be excluded. It comes as no surprise that a society focused on being young, dynamic, and "in control" is at a loss where ageing is concerned (pp. 109–110).

In a highly relevant and timely book, *What is the Good Life?* Luc Ferry (2005) has done a superb job in capturing the philosophical dilemmas of our modern era where technology has given us the tools to consider a personal transcendence—the maximal intensification of one's own existence quite independent from any historical or previous transcendent principles found in cosmic, religious or utopian philosophies (see also Said 2006). Yet this new metamorphosis of existence, this reliance on technology to cure and offer salvation has its costs,

> Quite comprehensively, this technological perspective encourages (and even renders obligatory) a veritable cult of performance for its own sake, thus shattering the old logic of meaning in favor of an exclusive use of the logic of competition. The historical processes that affect our daily lives, which are mechanically induced and elude the control of nation-states more and more each day, are developing at a speed that is undoubtedly accelerating but, above all, is subject to no visible purpose. In this perspective, to live, to survive, and to succeed become terms that are in the final analysis, synonymous: no matter what the "good life" might have meant in past times, it is now forced to give way to the "successful life"—or to a failed life. As a consequence… the principal menace burdening existence (aside from the fact that it comes to an end) resides in insignificance, banality, and ennui. (p. 11)

Ferry (2005) has insightfully analyzed the role of the "birth of science" and the "disenchantment of the world" as influential factors in driving the relentless pursuit of material gains and a loss of transcendental ideals to serve as compass points for human existence (see also Taylor 2007). One of the consequences of this philosophical vacuum is the allure of a more personal transcendence that seeks to escape our world with all of its flaws and imperfections via the tools of technology, which may offer eternal youth and immortality. We think it is extremely important to have teachers and students consider the longevity revolution, the SENS and SENSE models, and the role of anti-ageing medicine in the context of human motivations, insecurities, fears, and values that relate to happiness, salvation, time, and mortality, and "What is the good life?" and "Is it good enough?" (see Ryff and Singer 2008). More importantly, we need to revisit deeper questions that Cole and Winkler (1994) have already alluded to in their wonderful compilation, *The Oxford Book of Ageing*,

> Does ageing have an intrinsic purpose? Is there anything really important to be done after children are raised, jobs left, careers completed? Is old age the culmination of life? Does it contain potential for self-completion? What are the avenues for spiritual growth in later life? What are the roles and responsibilities of older people? What are the particular strengths and virtues of old age? Is there such a thing as a "good" old age? (p. 3)

As we enter into the second decade of the 21st century (and some 20 years after their publication), it appears that scientific research and medical technology has continued to alter the possibilities of human life to the point where some believe that "living within limits" is exactly what shall be overcome through the technological prowess of researchers who see the both the fountain of youth and the holy grail wrapped up into one big bioengineering project that is SENS or SENSE—or both—in our post ageing era (Critser 2010; Weiner 2010). And perhaps it is also time at this point in our historical moment to contemplate a new edition of the *Oxford Book of Ageing* that will capture both the classical reflections on the journey of life, but also welcome the reflections of modern scholars who weave philosophical threads into the technological advancements that alter the course of the ageing process itself (see Partridge et al. 2009). The questions posed by Cole and Winkler (1994) are still relevant today, but would the answers be any different than they were in 1994? *Is there such a thing as a "good" old age?* Exactly. The answers given by de Grey or Rose or by many of the transhumanists would shock and surprise many in the field of gerontology who suppose *ageing* is the very gift and reward for having lived so long. But whereas Petrarch, Shakespeare, and Montaigne reflected on ageing and found it wanting in many different ways, de Grey and Rose are no longer willing to simply reflect—*they want to do something about it.* And that passion, that conviction, is seemingly driven by the perspective that there are *no redeeming qualities* to ageing, but it is simply getting old, with all the attendant miseries of frailty. But it is more than just that. There are enormous social and medical costs associated with the biological ageing process and these costs will rise dramatically in the coming decades. And in response to this challenge a list of "biogerontology heavyweights" (as De Grey 2010, calls them in the collective sense) have written a compelling report that proposes a global initiative to translate recent research findings into interventions for ageing humans (Rae et al. 2010). One of the three proposed interventions that the group (Rae et al. 2010) highly recommends for immediate implementation is in the domain of regenerative medicine, including the bioengineering dimension and the related GRIN technologies.

We are not convinced that the single-minded obsession with defeating ageing by using bioengineering strategies at full speed ahead *without a deeper reflection process and philosophical discourse* is the path that we—in the larger collective social-cultural domain—should take if we are to embrace the GRIN technologies in the post ageing era. We should act, but we should do so fully conscionable and integrated into the fabric of the larger context of humanity who may or may not agree with the goals and perspectives of post ageing. For many people, embracing technology is *not* the way to "outlive the self" (see Kotre 1996) or engage the "commanding self" (see Shah 1994), or even experience a "gerotranscendent self" (Hyse and Tornstam 2009). We therefore submit that technology without philosophical embeddings is a simply a "tool"—and so are those who subscribe to it, as though "it" were the only important thing in solving the matters of life. We are *not* suggesting that Aubrey de Grey needs a refresher course in the writings of Kierkegaard ("The Sickness Unto Death"), or that Michael Rose should become more acquainted with Epictetus ("The Art of Living"), or that The American Academy of Anti-Ageing Medicine (A4M) could have invited both Szymborska (1995) and Kaja Silverman (2009) as their next keynote speakers, or that the transhumanists should consider the aesthetics of Shakespeare, which in large part hinge on the dynamics of time and ageing (see Charney 2009); we are primarily thinking about *the rest of us*: we who would have to live (perhaps "forever") with the consequences of any radical evolution altering the life course which now assumes limits.

But humanity *unlimited* changes the rules of the game. GRIN technologies that operate in a vacuum and are left unreflected upon are a foolish act of hubris affecting both the technologists and the multitude of humans interconnected through varied economic and environmental threads. Some, like de Grey, may disagree. He may see even see the call for an active philosophical engagement as interference and as a frivolous exercise. But we would counter that objection and ask both de Grey, and you the reader, and students in our classrooms: Whether or not we want to live longer, what is the point? Why live at all? What will a thousand years bring you that one hundred could not? Ageing has ended—now what? We submit that technology may change the *dimension of time* for such reflections, but we still (and believe that others also would) grapple with the existential reflections (see Hoffman 2009; Krueger 2009). We are right back to Camus and *The Myth of Sisyphus* where "Judging whether life is or is not worth living amounts to answering the fundamental question of philosophy" (see also Gems 2003). In fact, some may even find solace and transcendental significance in mortality and finitude. Consider this perspective by Silverman (2009) who examined the role of correspondences among human relations vis-à-vis works of art and literature, past and future, and how the "stories" connect us all.

> Finitude is the capricious and enabling of the attributes we share with others, because unlike the particular way in which each us looks, thinks, walks, and speaks, that connects us to a few other beings, it connects us to *every* other being. Since finitude marks the point where we end and others begin, spatially and temporally, it is also what makes room for them—and acknowledging these limits allows us to experience the expansiveness for which we year, because it gives us a powerful sense of our emplacement within a larger Whole. (p. 4)

We also submit that a deeper philosophical examination will help illuminate the motivations and values that influence the investigators and technicians involved the scientific (and non-scientific) endeavors in radical post ageing. The goal here is not for philosophy to serve as psychoanalysis or to instigate argumentum ad hominem; rather, the purpose is to engage both argument and explanation in order to explore the "idea" of science. We agree with Tauber (2009) that, "Science, as an epistemology, remains inextricably coupled to the existential questions that define human self-knowledge and understanding. That coupling deserves special scrutiny" (p. 36).

Thus, we are suggesting that for every book chapter or research article published on technology and ageing and set up as required reading in our classrooms as indicators of what the future may unveil for us, we should also consider as pedagogical "equal time" for book chapters and research articles that examine "Death and Dying in Anxious America" (Scheper-Hughes 2010), and the nuances of "happiness" (Diener and Biswas-Diener 2008) that influence an "American Mania" (Whybrow 2005), or challenge the notion that we are even well-equipped to find happiness at all (Haybron 2008), or that it is "overrated" (Belliotti 2004), or it is incorrectly measured in the first place (Krueger 2009), or counterproductive (Ehrenreich 2009), and that at best we "stumble our way to happiness" (Gilbert 2006). Technology may change our lives in many ways, but it may not offer or provide any magic solutions to perennial questions that relate to "the good life" or even how to "age well" (seeFischer et al. 2008; Franklin 2010; Krause 2009; Ostow 2009; Ryff and Singer 2008; Valliant 2002). Many of the scholars and advocates in the radical version of post ageing appear to want to leapfrog past these existential touchstones and jump headfirst into a brave new world that assumes the maps for the "traditional" journey of life (see Cole 1992; Smelser 2009) are simply archaic vestiges of the past and are no longer necessary templates for post-adolescence, as adulthood will seemingly become "different" in the era of post ageing and transhumanism.

In effect, we have indicated the materialization of the inflection point for *post ageing* and its utter dependence on the emergence of technologies to change the direction—and purpose—of the life course, but we also now propose that we will have come full circle by re-establishing the need for a dedicated and deep process of reflection in our educational venues (see Macilwain 2009). We submit that the presence of *ageing as a reflection* is a necessary condition to fully comprehend the significance of the ageing process itself both within the post ageing curvature (knowing full well that the goal of post ageing is to make ageing an *artifact*—to *end it*—and as a result we do not even have to think or reflect upon it at all). We also posit that ageing with reflection is an essential outside-looking-in optic in the modern milieu of this century where we have all but embraced the technological as manifested by both moderate and radical versions as *fait accompli* in human development in the 21st century—for better or for worse. We are also at a point where the prospect of *ending ageing* is no longer in the realm of fantastical mythology, but entirely technologically possible. In fact, the potential of immortality has become the central topic for several scholarly journal publications and grist for the blog mills that elevate technology and transhumanism as the desired future for humanity. But we, the jury, must convene and deliberate before we can reach the final verdict on this inflection point that is *post ageing*.

We have analyzed a great number of books and research articles, web sites and blog postings in order to survey the landscape for the intersection of technology and ageing, and we are strongly convinced that the *post ageing* era is upon us. As gerontologists and professionals invested in developing a relevant and viable curriculum for future leaders in the field of ageing, we are obligated to weave the various manifestations of technologies that intersect with the ageing process—including the emergent radical versions of post ageing that, in effect, seek to end the ageing process—along with any experiential discovery of what it is like to be an ageing being. Thus, the phenomenology of ageing is at stake in the full expression of the radical version of post ageing. But as we have seen, to some the end of ageing would be seen as the ultimate measure of success with technological advancements, a sure sign of victory against the attributes of senescence, typically portrayed as negative. In other words, there apparently is not much to be gained in experiencing the ageing process when the ultimate outcome is supposedly illness, suffering, decline, and inevitably, death. At best, it seems that the most we can do is to treat the symptoms, describe the challenges to social and government structures, and hope to compress morbidity the very ends of human limits in terms of natural life span. And for many, this is enough. This is sufficient given our resources, our ethics, and our needs and wants. We all want to live life to the maximum—optimally. If decline and frailty enter our existence, then so be it, but at least the presence of disease and decline would coincide in close proximity to the wall of limits. Natural limits. Life limited, but life lived fully in the longevity revolution.

For others that is grossly insufficient. Nor is it acceptable given the tools at our command. For some, technology (i.e., the GRIN technologies) is the solution to the problem of ageing; more so, it is the key to unlocking the limits of human life, opening up and making accessible an entire life experience beyond the so-called natural life span (see Gems 2003). The longevity revolution should not stop at a "natural" limit. There is no limit that is "natural" anymore. Being human and becoming an ageing individual is not a given and we should certainly not accept the compression of morbidity or optimal ageing as the final goal worthy of all of our efforts in gerontology and geriatrics. It is as though *ageing* is the touchstone by which we can determine whether or not we shall perhaps fully enhance the state of being human so that we might transcend ourselves into something greater—*better*. The experience of ageing is seen as robbing us of our full potential. If ageing were defeated, then by extension, the defeat of death would be the next "intervention." And both are highly interconnected in this regard; one could be immortal, but to age indefinitely ironically conjures up the Greek myth of Tithonus nightmarish condition, granted immortality by Zeus at the request of Eos who forgot to ask for eternal youth for her lover (see also Baltes 2006). It also relates to the Cumean Sybil, who, although she was a mortal, lived to about a thousand years. This came about when Apollo offered to grant her a wish in exchange for her virginity; she took a handful of sand and asked to live for as many years as the grains of sand she held. Later, after she refused the god's love, he allowed her body to wither away because she failed to ask for eternal youth. Her body grew smaller with age and eventually was kept in a jar, which was referenced by T.S. Eliot at the beginning of his masterpiece, *The Waste Land*.

How appropriate…*The Waste Land*. The verse and imagery conjure up the worst kind of condition of living…and living…and living in "a jar", where neither the person nor the contexts are able to make meaning, whether it is a hundred years or a thousand. The future of ageing is indeed biotechnological. But shall it also be philosophical? We have strongly indicated that post ageing should be embedded in the aesthetical, phenomenological, and hermeneutical—even when purists, advocates, and devotees of the GRIN technologies see no need to taint "the nature of technology" with any other perspective.

And there are signs that the examination of technology with ageing is receiving scholarly consideration from an interdisciplinary perspective as in the series of articles associated with the journal *Society*, and a symposium on the topic of "extending life indefinitely" (see Cohen 2009; Goodman 2009; Jasanoff 2009; and Kaye 2009), and in a special issue of *Medicine Studies* (Kampf and Botelho 2009) on the topic of anti-ageing and biomedicine which took a decidedly interdisciplinary approach to the topic. In a new book edited by Fahy et al. (2010), *The Future of Ageing*, there are at least twenty chapters that address the landscape of pathways to human life extension, but only one or two that even remotely address why we should extend human life *beyond limits*. We still have a ways to go, but that will be the task for each of us associated with the field of gerontology.

We propose that we are all, like Siddhartha Gautama, in the position of again confronting the three aspects of human life (old age, sickness, and death) that should serve to change us profoundly—and to begin the search for a lifetime. But in the post ageing era, we also need to reflect upon the potential for a new transformation via the GRIN technologies that would seek to alter all three aspects *in our lifetime*. We may wish for the longevity revolution, but we should also be *carefully* aware of what we wish for.

References

Arthur, W. B. (2009). *The nature of technology—What it is and how evolves*. New York: Free Press.

Atala, A., Lanza, R., Thomson, J., & Nerem, R. (Eds.). (2010). *Foundations of regenerative medicine*. San Diego, CA: Academic Press (Elsevier).

Baars, J. (2010). Philosophy of ageing, time, and finitude. In T. Cole, R. Ray, & Kastenbaum, R. (Eds.), *A guide to humanistic studies in ageing* (pp. 105–120). Baltimore MD: The Johns Hopkins University Press.

Baggini, J., & Fosl, P. (2010). *The philosopher's toolkit: A compendium of philosophical concepts and methods*. Malden, MA: Wiley-Blackwell.

Baltes, P. (2006). Facing our limits: Human dignity in the very old. *Daedalus, 135*, 32–39 (Winter).

Barzun, J. (2000). *From dawn to decadence: 1500 to the present*. New York: HarperCollins Publishers.

Bauerlein, M. (2008). *The dumbest generation: How the digital age stupefies young Americans and Jeopardizes our future*. London: Penguin Group.

Berger, T. W., & Glanzman, D. (Eds.). (2005). *Toward replacement parts for the brain: Implantable biomimetic electronics as neural prostheses*. Cambridge, MA: The MIT Press.

Bell, G., & Gemmell, J. (2009). *Total recall: How the e-memory revolution will change everything*. New York: Dutton.

Belliotti, R. A. (2004). *Happiness is overrated*. Lanham, MD: Rowman & Littlefield Publishers Inc.

Bowman, J. (2008). Is stupid making us google? *The New Atlantis, 22*, 75–80 (Summer).

Brodsky, C. (2009). *In the place of language: Literature and the architecture of the referent*. New York: Fordham University Press.

Brooks, S. (2010). The soul of the scientist of man. *The New Atlantis: A Journal of Technology & Society, 26*, 98–107 (Fall/Winter).

Brynjolfsson, E., & Saunders, A. (2010). *Wired for innovation: How technology is reshaping the economy*. Cambridge, MA: The MIT Press.

Carr, N. (2008). Is google making us stupid? What the internet is doing to our brains. *The Atlantic* (July/August). http://www.theatlantic.com/doc/200807/google.

Cascio, J. (2009). Technology: Get smart. *The Atlantic, 304*, 94–100.

Charney, M. E. (2009). Problematic of technology and the realms of salvation in Heidegger's philosophy. *Forum Philosophicum, 14*, 343–367.

Clark, A. (2007). Re-inventing ourselves: The plasticity of embodiment, sensing, and mind. *Journal of Medicine and Philosophy, 32*, 263–282.

Clark, A. (2010). *Supersizing the mind: Embodiment, action, and cognitive extension (philosophy of the mind)*. New York: Oxford University Press.

Cohen, E. (2009). The phenomenon of death. *Society, 46*, 221–223.

Cole, T. R. (1992). *The journey of life: A cultural history of ageing in America*. New York: Cambridge University Press.

Cole, T. R., Ray, R., & Kastenbaum, R. (2010). *A guide to humanistic studies in ageing*. Baltimore, MD: The Johns Hopkins University Press.

Cole, T. R., & Winkler, M. G. (Eds.). (1994). *The Oxford book of ageing: Reflections on the journey of life*. New York: Oxford University Press.

Cooper, A. (2009). Computing the cost: Nicholas Carr on how the internet is rewiring our brains. *The Sun, 49*, 4–11.

Costa, G. D. N. (Trans.). (2005). *Seneca: On the shortness of life*. New York: Penguin Books. (Original work published 56 A. D.).

Critser, G. (2010). *Eternity soup: Inside the quest to end ageing*. New York: Harmony Books.

Davenport, W. (1970). *The one culture*. New York: Pergamon Press.

De Grey, A. D. N. J. (2010). Reaping the longevity dividend in time: Biogerontology heavyweights advocate seeking late-onset interventions against ageing. *Rejuvenation Research, 13*(4), 383–384.

Deneen, P. J. (2010). Science, the humanities, and the university. *The New Atlantis: A Journal of Technology & Society, 26*, 60–68 (Fall/Winter).

Diener, E., & Biswas-Diener, R. (2008). *Happiness: Unlocking the mysteries of psychological wealth*. Malden, MA: Blackwell Publishing.

Dummett, M. (2010). *The nature and future of philosophy*. New York: Columbia University Press.

Ehrenreich, B. (2009). *Bright-sided: How the relentless promotion of positive thinking has undermined America*. New York: Metropolitan Books/Henry Holt and Company.

Eisele, T. D. (2009). *Bitter knowledge: Learning socratic lessons of disillusion and renewal*. Notre Dame, IN: Notre Dame University Press.

Fahy, G. M., West, M. D., Coles, L., & Harris, S. B. (Eds.). (2010). *The future of ageing: Pathways to human life extension*. New York: Springer.

Ferry, L. (2005). *What is the good life?*. Chicago, IL: University of Chicago Press.

Fillit, H., & Butler, R. N. (2009). The frail identity crisis. *Journal of American Geriatrics Society, 57*, 348–352.

Fischer, R., Norberg, A., & Lundman, B. (2008). Embracing opposites: Meanings of growing old as narrated by people aged 85. *International Journal of Human Development, 67*(3), 259–271.

Franklin, S. S. (2010). *The psychology of happiness: A good human life*. New York: Cambridge University Press.

Garreau, J. (2005). *Radical evolution: The promise and peril of enhancing our minds, our bodies—and what it means to be human*. New York: Broadway (Random House).

Gay, V. (2010). *Progress and values in the humanities: Comparing culture and science*. New York: Columbia University Press.

Gems, D. (2003, July–August). Is more life always better? The new biology and the meaning of life. Hastings Center Report, pp. 31–39.

Gilbert, D. (2006). *Stumbling on happiness*. New York: Alfred A Knopf.

Goodman, L. E. (2009). May you live to be 100! *Society, 46*, 240–246.

Hawkins, J. (2004). *Intelligence: How a new understanding of the brain will lead to the creation of truly intelligent machines*. New York: Times Books.

Haybron, D. M. (2008). *The pursuit of unhappiness: The elusive psychology of well-being*. New York: Oxford University Press.

Hoffman, E. (2009). *Time*. New York: Picador.

Hyse, K., & Tornstam, L. (2009). *Recognizing aspects of oneself in the theory of gerotranscendence*. Online publication from The Social Gerontology Group, Uppsala. http://www.soc.uu.se/research/gerontology/gerotrans.html.

Jasanoff, S. (2009). The past as prologue in life extension. *Society, 46*, 232–234.

Jones, R. (2004). *Soft machines: Nanotechnology and life*. New York: Oxford University Press.

Kagan, J. (2009). *The three cultures: Natural sciences, social sciences, and the humanities in the 21st century*. Cambridge, MA: Cambridge University Press.

Kampf, A., & Botelho, L. A. (2009). Anti-ageing and biomedicine: Critical studies on the pursuit of maintaining, revitalizing and enhancing ageing bodies. *Medicine Studies, 1*, 187–195.

Katz, S., & Peters, K. R. (2008). Enhancing the mind? Memory medicine, dementia, and the ageing brain. *Journal of Ageing Studies, 22*(348), 355.

Kaufman, S. (2010). The age of reflexive longevity: How the clinic and changing expectations of the life course are reshaping old age. In T. Cole, R. Ray, & R. Kastenbaum (Eds.), *A guide to humanistic studies in ageing: What does it mean to grow old?* (pp. 226–243). Baltimore, MD: The Johns Hopkins University Press.

Kaye, H. L. (2009). Death and us. *Society, 6*, 237–239.

Kenneally, I. (2010). The technocratic American university. *The New Atlantis: A Journal of Technology and Society*, 69–84 (Fall/Winter).

Kotre, J. (1996). *Outliving the self: How we live on in future generations*. New York: W.W. Norton & Co.

Krause, N. (2009). Meaning in life and mortality. *The Journals of Gerontology Series B: Psychological Sciences and Social Sciences, 64B*(4), 517–527.

Krueger, A. B. (2009). *Measuring the subjective well-being of nations: National accounts of time use and well-being*. Chicago: The University of Chicago Press.

Lawler, A. (2010, January/February). Tending the garden of technology. *Orion*, *29*, 36–41.

Macilwain, C. (2009). Watching science at work. *Nature, 464*(17), 840–842.

Manheimer, R. (2000). Ageing in the mirror of philosophy. In T. R. Cole, R. Kastenbaum, & R. E. Ray (Eds.), *Handbook of the humanities and ageing*. New York: Springer.

Mayer-Schonberger, V. (2009). *Delete: The virtue of forgetting in the digital age*. Princeton, NJ: Princeton University Press.

Ostow, M. (2009, June). What makes us happy? *The Atlantic*. http://theatlantic.com/doc/print/200906/happiness.

Partridge, B., Lucke, J., & Hall, W. (2009). Ethical, social, and personal implications of extended human lifespan identified by members of the public. *Rejuvenation Research, 12*(5), 351–357.

Pettman, D. (2006). *Love and other technologies: Retrofitting eros for the information age*. New York: Fordham University Press.

Plate, L., & Smelik, A. (Eds.). (2009). *Technologies of memory in the arts*. New York: Palgrave Macmillan.

Powers, W. (2010). *Hamlet's blackberry: A practical philosophy for building a good life in the digital age*. New York: HarperCollins.

Rae, M., Butler, R., Campisi, J., de Grey, A., Finch, C., & Gough, M., et al. (2010). The demographic and biomedical case for late-life interventions in ageing. *Science Translational Medicine*, *2*(40cm21), 1–6.

Reichle, I. (2009). *Art in the age of technoscience: Genetic engineering, robotics, and artificial life in contemporary art*. Wien, New York: Springer.

Rickman, H. (2004). *The riddle of the sphinx: Interpreting the human world*. Cranbury, NJ: Associated University Presses.

Ryff, C., & Singer, B. (2008). Know thyself and become what you are: A eudemonic approach to psychological well-being. *Journal of Happiness Studies, 9*, 13–29.

Said, E. W. (2006). *On late style: Music and literature against the grain*. New York: Pantheon Books.

Scheper-Hughes, N. (2010). Death and dying in anxious America. In H. Gusterson & C. Besteman (Eds.), *The insecure American: How we got here & what we should so about it* (pp. 317–344). Berkeley, CA: University of California Press.

Schulz, M. J., Shanov, V. N., & Yun, Y. (2009). *Nanomedicine; Design of particles, sensors, motors, implants, robots, and devices*. Boston, MA: Artech House.

Shah, I. (1994). *The commanding self*. London: The Octagon Press.

Silverman, K. (2009). *Flesh of my flesh*. Stanford, CA: Stanford University Press.

Small, H. (2007). *The long life*. Oxford: Oxford University Press.

Smelser, N. J. (2009). *The Odyssey experience: Physical, social, psychological, and spiritual journeys*. Berkeley, CA: University of California Press.

Snow, C. P. (1964). *The two cultures and a second look: An expanded version of the two cultures and the scientific revolution* (Canto Edition ed.). New York: Cambridge University Press.
Sorell, T. (1991). *Scientism: Philosophy and the infatuation with science*. New York: Routledge.
Specter, M. (2009). *Denialism: How irrational thinking hinders scientific progress, harms the planet, and threatens our lives*. New York: The Penguin Press.
Stenmark, M. (2001). *Scientism: Science, ethics and religion*. Burlington, VT: Ashgate Publishing.
Szymborska, W. (1995). *View with a grain of sand: Selected poems*. Boston, MA: Houghton Mifflin Harcourt.
Tauber, A. I. (2009). *Science and the quest for meaning*. Waco, TX: Baylor University Press.
Taylor, C. (2007). *A secular age*. Cambridge, MA: The Belknap Press of Harvard University Press.
Thagard, P. (2010). *The brain and the meaning of life*. Princeton, NJ: Princeton University Press.
Valliant, G. (2002). *Ageing well: Surprising guideposts to a happier life from the landmark harvard study of adult development*. Boston: Little Brown.
Vincent, J. (2006). Ageing contested: Anti-ageing science and the cultural construction of old age. *Sociology, 40*(4), 681–698.
Weiner, J. (2010). *Long for this world: The strange science of immortality*. New York: HarperCollins.
Whybrow, P. C. (2005). *American Mania: When more is not enough*. New York: W. W. Norton & Co.

Chapter 9
Longevity

Abstract We offer several issues for both argument and explanation at the intersection of philosophy and post ageing. Again, our goal here is to illustrate the fruitful exchange of philosophical concerns and the emergence of post ageing.

Kewords Biogerontology · Life extension · Prolongevity

So as we near the finish of this book we offer several issues for both argument and explanation at the intersection of philosophy and post ageing. These issues are clustered with several exemplars for two topics: (1) Longevity, which we will address in this chapter, and (2) Technology, which will be addressed in Chap. 10. Again, our goal here is to illustrate the fruitful exchange of philosophical concerns and the emergence of post ageing.

9.1 Meaning and Mortality

Krause (2009) found that older adults who have a strong sense of meaning in life are less likely to die over the course of the follow-up period than older people who do not have a strong sense of meaning in their lives. These results indicate the importance of meaning in the lives of older adults against the backdrop of "certain" death; that is, the certainty of mortality. Meaningfulness becomes meaningful to the mortal being. But what would be the significance of "meaning" in a life that is immortal, beyond ageing, transformed into a transhumanistic entity? Would the prospect of ending ageing change the significance of purpose in life?

K.F. Felsted and S.D. Wright, *Toward Post Ageing*,
Healthy Ageing and Longevity 1, DOI 10.1007/978-3-319-09051-1_9

9.2 Art and Humanities

At the intersection of the humanities and post ageing in terms of cultural and philosophical implications and understanding, Sachs (2010) offered an interesting interpretation for the creation of Beethoven's Ninth Symphony (*The Ninth Symphony and the World in 1824*). He wrote,

> If the Ninth Symphony's first movement is hurly-burly of the most horrific sort and the second a half-serious, half-playful battle, the third tells us that we have both lost and won–that, as aware human beings, we have no choice but to wade through the horror and anguish and die, but that we are able, from time to time, to see beyond and soar above these facts and to understand just enough to be able to appreciate the beauty of being mortal. After all, if anguish and death did not exist, art would not exist, nor would sensitivity to beauty. Or, to put a slightly different twists on an aphorism of Nietzsche's, sensitivity to beauty is one of our strongest defenses; without it, we would perish from truth" (pp. 144–145).

The implication of this perspective is that the dimension of art in the affairs of human existence owes its inspiration and creative catalyst to the awareness of mortality. The awareness and existential embrace of death is seen as a powerful motivator to the creative spirit; being mortal heightens the prospect of being sensitive to beauty and the sublime. This may be reflected in the art form of *vanitas* and *memento mori.* Although this interpretation of Sachs (2010) is debatable, it raises the question that if the goals of prolongevity, transhumanism, and perhaps immortality would be realized, how would this affect our understanding and appreciation for the artistic spirit in creation against the backdrop of a longer and longer duration of life? Will post ageing outcomes negate the drive and purpose of human artistic endeavors? Without finite limits to life, what would then be the point of "creativity"? How would the metaphysics of existence be affected? Would post ageing change the entire genre of literature, music and art, if the "tragic" limit of existence were to be transformed into living in perpetuity? Furthermore, this potential, this prospect, makes us wonder if then the Riddle of the Sphinx (which has been traditionally presented as, "Which creature in the morning goes on four legs, at mid-day on two, and in the evening upon three, and the more legs it has, the weaker it be?" Oedipus solved the riddle by answering, "Man—who crawls on all fours as a baby, then walks on two feet as an adult, and then walks with a cane in old age," may be rewritten into a new mythology for the era of post ageing. And so we present Oedipus Redux: "Which creature in the morning goes on four legs, at mid-day on two, and in the evening walks infinitely?" Our modern Oedipus now answers the riddle with, "Humans—who crawl on all fours as babies, then walk on two feet as adults, and then walk via virtual reality into the singularity."

9.3 Life Extension, Biomedical Research, and Ethical Concerns

There are perspectives from both sides of the argument that have addressed the "life extension project" based on philosophical examination and understanding. For example, Dumas and Turner (2007) have provided an extensive critique of biogerontology and have argued that biomedical research has potentially far greater negative consequences for the status of humans than what has been previously recognized. They offer interesting insights about the role of social justice and intergenerational inequalities should advances be realized in biogerontology. They propose that, "Once perceived as a vulnerable group and marginal group, the elderly may, through rejuvenation sciences, find themselves in serious inter-generational conflict with other social groups, especially with youth, who are a declining proportion of most populations" (p. 14). They are also critical of the field of sociology for not being more aware of these developments in biogerontology and summarize by noting that, "Living with prolongevity will require considerable changes to culture for which medicine has no answers" (p. 15). The co-author Turner (2009a) also has written the book, *Can We Live Forever? A Social and Moral Inquiry*, which examines the medical, cultural, religious and philosophical implications of life extension. Turner (2009b) was also a contributor to the special issue of *Society*, which published several reports based on the symposium, "Extending Life Indefinitely"; Turner proposed that the culture of the baby boomer generation would embrace the benefits of life extension because, "Death is no longer acceptable and ageing should be treated as a disease that is susceptible to medical treatment; indeed extending life is merely the extrapolation of current medical practice" (p. 259). Turner (2009b) went on say that we should try to distinguish between "living" and "surviving" since "the real issue is not whether technology or medical science can really deliver health longevity, but whether we can find any meaning in mere survival…the question of living (not surviving) raises moral and religious issues that science cannot (and does not aim) to solve" (p. 260). While some have debated the existential undesirability of immortality due to "boredom" (Bortolotti and Nagasawa 2009) or the distribution of health care resources for increasing life spans (Farrant 2009), or the Malthusian versus Methuselah choice (Davis 2005; Gavrilov and Gavrilov 2010), it is the work of Temkin (2008), "Is Living Longer Living Better?" a paper in the *Journal of Applied Philosophy*, that brings to the forefront of discussion a deeper examination of the prospects for living longer (but perhaps not better). Temkin stated that,

> Indeed, I think they are sufficiently worrisome that we should think long and hard about supporting longevity research that might ultimately end ageing. I do not okay this lightly. As indicated previously, I subscribe to the Enlightenment project of science ameliorating the human condition. The last thing I favour is Philosophy standing in the way of human progress. But the stakes in this area are so huge that it is imperative to carefully determine whether stopping ageing really *would* be progress. And I fear we must have this debate *before* the research goes too far. After all given our powerful fear of death, and the overwhelming human propensity to use whatever technologies become available, it is almost certain that any anti-ageing technology that is developed *will* be used once it becomes available. And make no mistake, once research points the way to feasible anti-ageing technology such technology *will* become available (p. 208).

References

Bortolotti, L., & Nagasawa, Y. (2009). Immortality without boredom. *Ratio, 22*, 262–272.

Davis, J. K. (2005). Life-extension and the Mathusian objection. *Journal of Medicine and Philosophy, 30*, 27–44.

Dumas, A., & Turner, B. S. (2007). The life extension project: A sociological critique. *Health Sociology Review, 16*, 5–17.

Farrant, A. (2009). The fair innings argument and increasing life spans. *Journal of Medical Ethics, 35*, 53–56.

Gavrilov, L. A. & Gavrilov, N. S. (2010). Demographic consequences of defeating ageing. *Rejuvenation Research, 3*(2). Retrieved at: http://liebertonline.com/doi/abs/10.1089/rej.2009.0977

Krause, N. (2009). Meaning in life and mortality. *The Journals of Gerontology Series B: Psychological Sciences and Social Sciences, 64B*(4), 517–527.

Sachs, H. (2010). *The ninth: beethoven and the world in 1824*. New York: Random House.

Temkin, L. S. (2008). Is living longer living better? *Journal of Applied Philosophy, 25*(3), 193–210.

Turner, B. S. (2009a). *Can we live forever? a sociological and moral inquiry*. New York: Anthem Press.

Turner, B. S. (2009b). Longevity ancient and modern. *Society, 46*, 255–261.

Chapter 10
Technology

Abstract This raises challenging questions about the role of forgetting and remembering in the lives of older adults and a debate about if both are important—or is one more important to well-being than the other and what role should technology play in supplementing creating autobiographies and enhancing the practice of reminiscence and story-telling? What role will technology play in the interventions for those older adults with cognitive impairments? What are the ethical and legal issues that surround "perfect remembering" due to digital technologies? Perfect remembering—or that lack of forgetting—has interesting implications for research in our field where the cognitive capacity to remember (and function accordingly) and the fear of forgetting loom large in our literature.

Keywords Assistive healthcare robots · Cognitive extension · Embodied mind · Memory and technology · Technogenesis · Technological memes · Temes

10.1 Memory and Forgetting

In the book, by Mayer-Schonberger (2009), *Delete: The Virtue of Forgetting in the Digital Age*, there are concerns about the prospect of "perfect remembering" in the digital age. Mayer-Schonberger offers a provocative counter argument that,

> …forgetting performs an important function in human decision-making. It permits us to generalize and abstract from individual experiences. It enables us to accept that humans, like all life, changes over time. It thus anchors us to the present, rather than keeping us tethered permanently to an ever more irrelevant past. Plus, forgetting empowers societies to be forgiving to its members, and to remain open to change. Digital remembering undermines the important role forgetting performs, and thus threatens us individually and as a society in our capacity to learn, to reason, and to act in time. It also exposes us to a potentially devastating human over-reaction–a complete disregard of our past (pp. 197–198).

This raises challenging questions about the role of forgetting and remembering in the lives of older adults and a debate about if both are important—or is one more important to well-being than the other and what role should technology play in

K.F. Felsted and S.D. Wright, *Toward Post Ageing*,
Healthy Ageing and Longevity 1, DOI 10.1007/978-3-319-09051-1_10

supplementing creating autobiographies and enhancing the practice of reminiscence and story-telling? What role will technology play in the interventions for those older adults with cognitive impairments? What are the ethical and legal issues that surround "perfect remembering" due to digital technologies? Perfect remembering—or that lack of forgetting—has interesting implications for research in our field where the cognitive capacity to remember (and function accordingly) and the fear of forgetting loom large in our literature. This topic has also received the attention of philosophers such as Alexander (2009) who used the short story by F. Scott Fitzgerald, "The Curious Case of Benjamin Button," to examine both the ethical and moral consequences of "forgetting" as a result of the "grotesque phenomenon" of Button's chronological and bodily ages running in different directions. Even though the story (and the movie directed by David Fincher in 2008) is fictional, it serves as a backdrop for exploring the dimensions of having chronological age severed from psychological age, having the human experience be transformed whether in the imagination of artists or by bioengineers and those interested in rejuvenation medicine and those who espouse prolongevity–and immortality. In this case, Alexander (2009) points to the impact of forgetting and the role of memory in human development,

> Benjamin Button's life evokes awareness of the breakdown of such levels of importance and of their various claims to a place in memory. His life stresses the disruption and havoc that can emerge when the threads of memory are severed from salient features of a life. It brings out how such severance is an obstacle to change. And by contrast it brings out equally and vividly–what we may have failed to notice because so evident–namely, the importance of threads of memory to the significance that a person can find in life. By highlighting forgetfulness damages and dissipates Benjamin Button's topsy-turvy existence, we can grasp how forgetfulness may overlap into moral concerns (p. 16).

10.2 Reverse Engineering the Brain

In an article in the journal, *Biomedical Computation*, (pp. 10–17) on the topic of computer consciousness, the author Friedman (2009) interviewed several researchers who collectively believe that "mind" arises from the "wetware" that is the brain, and they proclaimed that the best way to create mind-like intelligence into machines is to reverse engineer the structure, function, and dynamics of the brain. One researcher, Gerald Edelman (Director of the Neurosciences Institute and chair of neurobiology at the Scripps Research Institute in San Diego, California) indicated the goal was to craft a conscious artifact. Edelman says, "Philosophers have owned the field of consciousness research from time immemorial. What could be more romantic, remarkable or valuable, than to take on their quest?" Should this be the goal and quest of brain researchers–to create a mind-like machine? To create a conscious artifact? One of the purported benefits of this technological goal would be that brain scientists hope to simulate the effect of strokes, tumors, or neurological disorders such as Alzheimer's or Parkinson's disease to understand how they derail brain dynamics. Do these potential benefits outweigh any concerns about blurring the boundary of consciousness and what defines "us" as humans?

10.3 Embodied Minds, Ageing, and Technology

Lakoff and Johnson (1999) have proposed a provocative perspective in the use of philosophical inquiry in advancing the notion that when we ask philosophical questions, "we use a reason shaped by the body, a cognitive unconscious to which we have no direct access, and metaphorical thought of which we are largely unaware" (p. 7). That is to say, the tools of philosophical inquiry, such as concepts and reasons, are *embodied* and are the product of the body and architecture of the brain. Thus reasoning is not independent of the body (disembodied); it is very much brain and body dependent. So, in effect, philosophical inquiry (conceptual systems) is the result of body/brain interactions (perceptual and motor-systems). This line of thinking is similar to the work of Hannah and Maiese (2009) and their core ideas associated with Essential Embodiment Theory. But Clark (2010) has taken this perspective a step further (and made it perhaps even more provocative) by proposing a philosophical picture that extends the mind beyond the "brain-bound" and into the environment in which we interact. In other words, cognition leaks out into the body and the world. Thus, the perspective of cognitive extension and the possibility of human-machine interface and the role of biotechnologies integrated into body systems. This raises the possibility that (or at least a further examination of how) we might reexamine assistive technologies and gerotechnology as a part of the philosophical perspective of cognitive extension. We think there is the need to consider both the moderate and radical versions of post ageing within the perspectives of embodied minds and cognitive extension. This becomes especially important as we see emergent studies like the work of Buse (2010) who argued that although there is a growing body of research on the experiences of older Internet users, the embodiment dimension of these encounters with new technologies has yet to be examined in detail. Buse (2010) has emphasized the importance of situating computer use in alter life within people's biographical experiences of technology throughout the life course. Furthermore, as the inflection point of post ageing gains momentum toward the radical version, questions (and further examination) will be necessary in order to address the role of artificial intelligence, robotics, and the goals of transhumanism, in light of the moral use of technology (see Garvey 2007) and in context of Blackmore's (2010) intriguing proposal of "temes" (or "technological memes") which are considered to be digital information stored, copied, varied and selected by machines. Blackmore has stated that humans like to think they are the designers, creators and controllers of this newly emerging (technological) world but we are merely stepping stones from one replicator to the next.

10.4 Assistive Technology and Robots

The use of assistive robots in health care applications assumes the ageing process as a given in the human organism, but offers robotic technology as supplement to social care and monitoring strategies for the older adult in long term care facilities. The work by Nejat et al. (2010) raises the question and the need to further explore human–robot interactions and discuss the ethical issues involved with robots as supplementary–or even complementary–to human staffing in long term facilities. Some may argue this represents an abdication of the care ethic for older adults in our society, while others may see this as a necessary strategy for meeting the shortage challenges in nursing staff and the high rate of turnover in nursing assistants.

10.5 Cognitive Enhancements and Continuity or Discontinuity of "Self" in Post Ageing

Given the interest for many theorists in gerontology who have an interest in biological and environment influences on personality and on the qualitative and quantitative changes in the ageing person over time (e.g., life course studies and lifespan developmental psychology) and the several sociological theories associated with ageing (e.g., continuity theory) Schneider (2009) has proposed that that a key philosophical issue associated with transhumanism is the challenge of addressing the ontological issue of a continuous personal identity, specifically within the context of cognitive enhancement, such that after cognitive enhancements are implemented, there is much more that has changed than simply the addition of enhancements. Rather, one has to ask, "Will this radically enhanced creature still be me?" Another way of examining this issue is to consider the possibility of a demarcation point by which the original "you" is no longer you and is now a replicate of the former self due to significant changes in the self-state that the alteration takes place. That is, the "essential properties" of the self (the original you) are now replaced by modifications and interventions, and therefore, the new self is nothing like the old self, and thus raises the question: would you (the former self) then cease to exist? This issue sounds very much like the Ship of Theseus paradox from Plutarch's *Vita Thesei*, 22–23 (translated by Dryden; see Dryden (2014):

> The ship wherein Theseus and the youth of Athens returned had thirty oars, and was preserved by the Athenians down even to the time of Demetrius Phalereus, for they took away the old planks as they decayed, putting in new and stronger timber in their place, insomuch that this ship became a standing example among the philosophers, for the logical question of things that grow; one side holding that the ship remained the same, and the other contending that it was not the same.

Schneider (2009) argued that, "Without a firm handle on this issue, the transhumanist developmental trajectory is perhaps the technophile's alluring path to suicide." This relates to Roden's (2010) critical perspective of the speculative posthumanists (e.g., Vernor Vinge, Ray Kurzweil, and Hans Moravec) who claim, "that descendants of current humans could cease to be human by virtue of technical alteration" (p. 28). This then leads to another *related issue within this topic, the problematical process of* "knowing" what lies on the other side of transhumanism; in other words, we humans and transhumans may be capable of designing and organizing the right antecedents in place that can lead to the Singularity (or Methuselarity)—and thus posthuman alterity (the transcendence of posthumanism), but we may not be able to predict, or control, or understand, or even explain what the alterity is to be like (thus possibly anti-prognostic) given the human limitations associated with our finite cerebral capabilities and cognitive framework (Kantian noumena versus phenomena) that is selective and conditional. Roden (2010) has highlighted a unique philosophical conundrum with any discussion of human versus posthuman distinctions because any understanding of the postworld condition, which is presumably post singularity and post human, beyond morbidity and mortality, and quite possibly beyond the human characteristics of our own cognitive constraints. In effect, and philosophically speaking, posthumanism is essentially unknowable to us (as humans or as transhumans) and it is analogous to the Kantian *thing-in-itself* (noumena) whereby we cannot know of something that transcends the "principled limits of human cognition and knowledge" (Roden 2010, p. 20)—and instead all that we could possibly propose and fathom would be the representations of what we speculate are to be post human conditions (or sensory forms) given our Kantian cognitive constraints (time and space). Roden (2010) succinctly summarizes the conundrum in this fashion,

> Discounting the posthuman is morally irresponsible, though, given the possible role of transhumanist intervention in producing it. Thus transhumanists should try to evaluate the emergence of an incommensurate posthuman alterity. However, if we recognize evaluation as a non-starter, any attempt to do so would be incoherent. Thus it appears that transhumanists are morally obliged to evaluate the unevaluable. We can refer to this impossible demand as the 'posthuman impasse' (p. 29).

But Roden (2010) has offered a creative and viable alternative to the binary roles of *either human or post human*; we think that this perspective has promising affinity with our proposed inflection point of post ageing [5.x] and the *continuum of technological integration* with the ageing experience (moderate and radical version). We also think Roden's perspective of technogenesis brings to the forefront the nuances of the continuity or discontinuity of self with potential NBIC technologies. For example, whereas individuals like Kurzweil and de Grey have contemplated a critical juncture of human alterity (i.e., the singularity, methuselarity) where humans transcend their finite corporeal and finite existence via either machine or superlongevity strategies that involve an array of NBIC technologies, Roden (2010) proposes that the technology has always been a constant transformative process in the evolutionary process of humans, and that as

Andy Clark (2003) has stated, “We are already masters at incorporating nonbiological stuff and structure deep into our physical and cognitive routines” (p. 142). In other words, humans are already “natural born cyborgs” and that, via technogenesis, the use of technology is very much a part of our human nature (see also Taylor 2010). The impact of this perspective is that our minds (our cognitive abilities) are seen extended across the body and into the environment (see “Supersizing the Mind,” Clark 2010) and beyond the human “self” such that technology becomes an “exo-self.” Here the orientation is not so much a transformation from human/transhuman to a definitive and critical threshold that creates an all-together different “post human” due to technological interventions, rather, technology is a matter of degree such that body and extra-body interactions are seamless and permeable and create a “flat ontology.” According to Roden (2010), the future is less post human—and more of a deepening hybrid of human-machine integration—a proliferation of cyborg evolutionary potential where technology and human interactions are highly interwoven. The essence of human*ness* is preserved, but nevertheless changed dramatically.

References

Alexander, H. (2009). Reflections on Benjamin button. *Philosophy and Literature, 33*, 1–17.

Blackmore, S. (2010). The third replicator. *New York Times*. Retrieved from August 22, 2010, from http://opinionator.blogs.nytimes.com/2010/08/22/the-third-replicator/

Buse, C. E. (2010). E-scaping the ageing body? Computer technologies and embodiment in alter life. *Ageing and Society, 30*, 987–1009.

Clark, A. (2003). *Natural born Cyborgs: Minds, technologies, and the future of human intelligence*. New York: Oxford University Press.

Clark, A. (2010). *Supersizing the mind: Embodiment, action, and cognitive extension (Philosophy of the mind)*. New York: Oxford University Press.

Dryden, J. (2014). *Vita thesei* [Trans.] (22–23). Retrieved from http://classics.mit.edu/Plutarch/theseus.html (see also https://faculty.washington.edu/smcohen/320/theseus.html)

Friedman, R. (2009). Reverse engineering the brain. *Biomedical Computation, 5*, 10–17.

Garvey, J. (2007). The moral use of technology. *Royal Institute of Philosophy Supplement, 82*, 241–260.

Hannah, R., & Maiese, M. (2009). *Embodied minds in action*. New York: Oxford University Press.

Lakoff, G., & Johnson, M. (1999). *Philosophy in the flesh: The embodied mind and its challenge to western thought*. New York: Basic Books (Perseus Book Groups).

Mayer-Schonberger, V. (2009). *Delete: The virtue of forgetting in the digital age*. New Jersey: Princeton University Press.

Nejat, G., Nies, M., & Sexton, T. R. (2010). An interdisciplinary team for the design and integration of assistive robots in health care applications. *Home Health Care Management and Practice, 22*(2), 104–110.

Roden, D. (2010). Deconstruction and excision in philosophical posthumanism. *Journal of Evolution and Technology, 21*(1), 27–36.

Schneider, S. (2009). *Mindscan: Transcending and enhancing the human brain*. Retrieved September 8, 2010, from http://www.sas.upenn.edu/~sls/documents/Schneider-Mindscanproofs.pdf

Taylor, T. (2010). *The artificial ape: How technology changed the course of human evolution*. New York: Palgrave Macmillian.

Chapter 11
Philosophical Antecedents for Post Ageing

Abstract We propose that a significant part of post ageing is therefore revolutionary and heterodoxy and iconoclastic if taken from the stance of the established domain and received view of gerontology. We further propose that there is need for the renaissance of an active philosophical examination of the emergence of post ageing scholarship activities. Whether or not one side can convince the other or win the hearts and minds of the general public, the post ageing inflection point has indeed occurred and there is the need to utilize the full range of philosophical tools at hand (e.g., epistemology, ontology, ethics) to understand the underpinnings of how it came to be, and where it is leading us.

Keywords Gerontology and philosophy · Gerontology and technology · Postageing · Posthumanism · Transcendence · Transhumanism

The story of Prince Siddhārtha (who later became Gautama Buddha) and his exposure to the "four sights" is known to many individuals, and we think it is an excellent story to indicate the modern crossroads for the integration of gerontology, technology, and philosophy. If you recall, the "four sights"—an old man, a sick man, a corpse and an ascetic—were instrumental in changing the course of Prince Siddhārtha's life journey—and his goal to address the challenges of existence is a world of suffering, disease, and death. Before witnessing firsthand the four sights, he had been confined to his palace by his father, who feared that he would become an ascetic if he came into contact with sufferings of life according to a prediction. However, on his first venture out of the palace with his charioteer Channa, he observed four sights and these observations affected him deeply and made him realize the sufferings of all beings, and compelled him to begin his spiritual journey. The journey led to important principles and practice that would allow individuals to escape the fate of suffering and death. The desire to respond to the challenges of life—including disease, ageing, and death—has been the lifeblood of many philosophical writings over the course of many centuries and some approaches are passive, some active, some life-affirming, some transcendental, and some utopian, and some dystopian. But in our contemporary time and place into the second decade of the 21st century, we are again like Prince Siddhārtha

K.F. Felsted and S.D. Wright, *Toward Post Ageing*,
Healthy Ageing and Longevity 1, DOI 10.1007/978-3-319-09051-1_11

confronting the "four sights"—an old man, a sick man, a corpse and an ascetic—in the sense that we too face a momentous crossroads of choices that reflect decisions in regards to ageing and mortality. But this time—and this place—the tools, the principles, and the practice are associated with techné, techtonics, or technogenesis, or the technosphere, or GRIN, or NBIC, and again we are in the position to choose a path to address the very same four sights we see before us: Can we conquer disease? Can we end ageing? Can we escape death? Do we need any metaphysical or spiritual guidance and direction in these matters? Many would argue that the answers are directly in front of us and the path is clearly marked with technological interventions such that disease, ageing, and death can be eliminated. They would continue that the only asceticism needed is the realization that the transcendental experience of humans leading the way—as transhumanists—to the possible domain of post humanism is our quest—and our duty is to act, solve the problem, design the technology, to "just do it"—without regard to ontological or ethical debate. This has also led to a plethora of neologisms that try to capture the domain of technological interventions on both sides such as death hackers, the immortalists, deathists and so on. Evidently we have even reached a point where one transhumanist, Ben Goertzel (2010), has written a practical philosophy for the posthuman era titled, *A Cosmist Manifesto.* It is remarkable that in our time and place we can even contemplate ageing as "optional", as a conscious choice to bypass and then surpass. But such is the prospect of a *post ageing* inflection point. We have proposed that the field of ageing has entered into a new inflection point known as post ageing, which is the result of not only the use of advanced technologies to intervene on behalf of the welfare of ageing individuals to enable and "age-in-place" (the moderate version), but also the aggressive efforts of using technologies to slow, or stop, or reverse the ageing process (the radical). This kind of intervention is vastly different in the sense that the goals are scientifically possible yet demand the scrutiny of why such endeavors should take place, and to what purpose and to what end are the interventions rationalized, and who are the proponents and opponents to post ageing activities. Post ageing represents a significant revolution of thought that no longer accepts ageing as a "given" outcome to human development. In other words, post ageing activities are not primarily engaged in *reflection*, or the viewpoint associated with seeing ageing as a biomedical problem so as to treat primary disease and sequela, or to engage in policy interventions that address the changes of demographic transitions. Nor is it to emphasize strategies that would maximize well-being for ageing individuals (optimal ageing)—because the above inflection points assume the ageing experience inevitable and axiomatic to the human condition. While it is possible to optimize the ageing experience through the compression of morbidity and the extension of life expectancy, post ageing's trajectory is toward escaping the ageing process altogether. In post ageing, the focus and actions are upon changing the ageing process, such that humans should use technology to the fullest extent to change the course of human development, so that either the effects of ageing are offset through technological means, or ageing is to be treated as though a disease, or the ageing individual is changed as an entity in need of avoiding the ageing process, and most dramatically that the ageing experience is to be transformed such that technology can become the mechanism to enable a transcendence away and above the corporeal and finite human condition that we have to come to associate (naturally) with decline—and morality. Post ageing, in its most radical manifestation, seeks to escape the fortunes for the second half of life, which many assume to be the domain of senescence, decline, and frailty. In contrast, post ageing is represented by the use of technology as the intervention to make ageing an artifact. In post ageing, to accept ageing as "inevitable" or "natural" would be an abdication of our supposed destiny to transcend our current state of existence. Within the sphere of anti-ageing medicine or transhumanism or rejuvenation medicine, ageing is the targeted barrier—the ultimate challenge—to ultimate fulfillment and supposed happiness.

Thus, senescence should be actively and intrusively altered, removed, and excised from the human experience, as it represents the underutilization of the human drive to overcome obstacles to progress and achievement (through science and technology), and accepting the status quo is tantamount to the acquiescence of failure. We propose that a significant part of post ageing is therefore revolutionary and heterodoxy and iconoclastic if taken from the stance of the established domain and received view of gerontology. We further propose that there is need for the renaissance of an active philosophical examination of the emergence of post ageing scholarship activities. But as we have already indicated, the philosophical examination of technology has already been proven to be fertile domains for scholarship. Take as an example the work of Charley (2009) who has examined the perspectives of technology based in Heidegger's philosophy and suggested that, "we can no longer look at technology in a neutral way, as a toy which we can play with without looking at the consequences of its use. Technology raises an ethical responsibility that we cannot evade" (p. 366). This represents an example of philosophical interest in technological developments in general—without specific regard for application to a period of life or necessarily as it may offer insights to ontological perspectives as an ageing individual.

We have also noted that the philosophical examination of ageing itself has also been proven to be fertile domain for scholarship—such as in the works of Cole et al. (2010)—but the two elements of ageing and technology *together*, especially in the radical version of post ageing, have rarely been pursued as viable philosophical areas for discourse. We think of the critical integration as *necessary* because post ageing should be subject to ethical examination, discursive scrutiny, hermeneutical analysis, and historiography, as post ageing involves humans driving the inflection point and humans as either the supposed beneficiaries or victims, and humans as the transition process that is leading to something quite transcendental—post humanism—if the technology as some envision were to proceed and be fulfilled. Such transitions have the human experience to negotiate with—and to understand more fully, especially as the post ageing inflection point has the potential to be a monumental shift in the ontological status of existence—of life.

In response to this assertion, we present an example of where the philosophy and post ageing have the potential to be integrated and then present specific nodes of philosophical inquiry to post ageing activities. Floridi (2009) has advanced a philosophy of information, within which he has proposed a "fourth revolution" in the historiography of science. The first three revolutions (Copernican, Darwinian, Freudian) created a process of dislocation and reassessment of humanity's fundamental nature and role in the universe, and the fourth revolution, related to *informational and computer technologies*, again modified our ontological perspectives. In other words, from Floridi's (2009) philosophical perspective, the (proposed) fourth revolution has forced us (once again) to consider that humans are informational organisms among many others, "significantly but not dramatically different from natural entities and agents and smart, engineered artifacts" (p. 156). This is a provocative thesis by Floridi who has elevated the impact of technology on par with the macro-level impact of discoveries associated with Copernicus, Darwin, and Freud. The epistemological and ontological ramifications are monumental if one ascribes to the notion that technology and information flow can be a seamless continuity between human and machine, as this changes the role of humans once again. And this is what we find fascinating with the advent of post ageing—that technology has altered our lives in fundamental ways and it represents the manifestation of the Floridi's (2009) fourth revolution into the domain of gerontology. The process of ageing, and the ageing experience, may never be the same again. But the post ageing inflection point has only recently emerged, and we are in the unique position to critically examine and evaluate the unfolding with philosophical perspectives. This is especially desired as post ageing captures not only the proponents and the advocates for transforming (ending) ageing but also the scholars who contest the scientific validity of such endeavors. But whether or not one side can convince the other or win the hearts and minds of the general public, the post ageing inflection point has indeed occurred and there is the need to utilize the full range of philosophical tools at hand (e.g., epistemology, ontology, ethics) to understand the underpinnings of how it came to be, and where it is leading us.

Thus, one of the alluring issues surrounding the prospects of a post ageing inflection point [5.x] is not only the potential for using a philosophical approach to analyze and understand the motivations and behaviors of the recognized leaders and advocates who pursue such activities when promoting and using nanotechnologies, robotics, artificial intelligence, and genomics to "enhance" human development, but also to determine if there are any philosophical perspectives that are purported to support, justify, lend credence to, or guide the trajectory of post ageing activities. Here we share with readers a distinct nodal perspective on the post ageing inflection point (with emphasis on the radical version) with a recommendation to examine potential philosophical underpinnings when examining the drives, the motivations, the intellectual as well as emotional catalysts for pursuing the biotechnological quest of transcending or overcoming the ageing experience.

In this case, the philosophical perspectives of Friedrich Nietzsche are brought into focus, in particular to the debate of whether Nietzsche's viewpoints support or negate the goals of transhumanism and in particular the notion of using technology to "create" a better more perfected human that transcends frailty, morbidity, and ultimately mortality—to the point by which humans are surpassed by a superhuman—the *Übermensch.* In the special issue of the *Journal of Evolution and Technology* (Vol. 21, Issue 1, 2010), the editor-in-chief Russell Blackford (2010) brings together an array of scholars to react and expand on an article, "Nietzsche, the Overman, and Transhumanism" by Stephan Lorenz Sorgner (2009) that had been published previously in the same journal. Sorgner had argued that there were significant *similarities* between the concept of the posthuman and Nietzsche's notion of the overhuman (aka the "overman" or "superman"). Several of the contributing authors, following the path of Bostrom (2005), such as Hauskeller (2010) and Hibbard (2010), disagreed with Sorgner's contention of the philosophical nuances of Nietzsche as influencing transhumanist ideas. Instead they believed that the proper antecedents to transhumanism should be associated with either the philosophies of J.S. Mills or Thomas Hobbes. Other contributors, such as More (2010), argue that Nietzsche directly influenced transhumanist ideas. Bainbridge (2010), though somewhat skeptical about Nietzsche's philosophical perspectives, discussed the possibility for technological transcendence in the near future. Bainbridge suggested that there are four possible routes over the abyss ("Man is a rope stretched between the animal and the Superman—a rope over an abyss") and toward the *Übermensch* (the overman): *biological transformation, computational transformation, psychotherapeutic transformation, and utopian transformation.* Bainbridge cleverly designates the biotechnology and computational technology as "Apollonian" routes to transcendence, while the psychotherapeutic and utopian have more in common with the "Dionysian" approach. Interestingly enough, Bainbridge (2010) suggested that the time for philosophizing about transhumanism was over, and it was time to *begin the journey* over the abyss toward the transcendental Overman via all four routes. But we think: *not so fast.*

The rush to find the philosophical antecedent in supporting the principles of transhumanism and posthumanism with historical figures such as Nietzsche is fraught with many problems: two of the most important ones being either that his writings have been misinterpreted or many of his concepts and principles run counter to the notion of a transcendental quest to overcome the ageing experience. The implications of Nietzsche's quest to counter nihilism, and the excesses of Platonism, and the decay of Christianity's template for answers to challenges of existential significance led to his call for a spiritual renewal—via the *Übermensch*—to a profoundly life-affirming choice to embrace the love of fate (amor fati)—the life that we have—with all of its sufferings and challenges—and yes, even the finality of death (Pippin 2010; Wicks 2007). Nietzsche did not necessarily promote a superman to avoid ageing and death; rather his writings indicate more of a superhuman strength (a new philosophy, a new spirituality, a new set of morals) to endure the daily grind of life—a life that is finite and one that you would gladly repeat over and over again (eternal recurrence). Nietzsche was against escapism via otherworldly beliefs or Platonic ideals; instead, his approach was about the unconditional acceptance of existence. Nietzsche would most likely find the transcendentalism associated with transhumanism via technological interventions foreign to his philosophical prescription of embracing life and carpe diem, and any suggestion for the *deification of foreverness* was simply not in his writings (see Pippin 2010; Wicks 2007).

In contrast with others who see Nietzsche's writings as an antecedent to transhumanism, we are more in agreement with Michael Ure (2009) who proposes a convincing argument that Nietzsche's philosophy (*amor fati*) has more in common with the Stoic school of school of philosophy than many have understood. And this brings us back full circle to the first inflection point of "ageing as reflection" where we first addressed the works of Marcus Aurelius ("Meditations") and Seneca. It seems to us that in the domain of post ageing that either we are ready to embrace *The Cosmist Manifesto* (Goertzel 2010) as the philosophical foundation for the future of post humanism or we are ready to *reconsider* the principles of Nietzsche—and the revival of wisdom found in the Stoic philosophy and its applications for modern society (Graver 2007; Irvine 2009)—and whether we live for a hundred years—or a thousand.

And with that caveat, we finish this book with an excerpt from one of the greatest writers of the 20th century, Jorge Luis Borges (Coleman 2000), and we hope you too will reflect upon his words as they apply to the remainder of this century..

> What is longevity? It is the horror of exiting in a human body whose faculties are in decline. It is insomnia measured by decades and not by metal hands. It is carrying the weight of the seas and pyramids, of ancient libraries and dynasties, of the dawns that Adam saw. It is being well aware that I am bound to flesh, to a voice I detest, to my name, to routinely remembering, to Castilian, over which I have no control, to feeling nostalgic for the Latin I do not know. It is trying to sink into death and being unable to sink into death. It is being and continuing to be. (p. 433)

References

Bainbridge, W. S. (2010). Burglarizing Nietzsche's tomb. *Journal of Evolution & Technology, 21*(1), 37–45.

Blackford, R. (2010). Editorial: Nietzsche and European posthumanisms. *Journal of Evolution & Technology, 21*(1), i–iii.

Bostrom, N. (2005). A history of transhumanist thought. *Journal of Evolution & Technology, 14*(1), 1–25.

Charley, M. E. (2009). Problematic of technology and the realms of salvation in Heidegger's philosophy. *Forum Philosophicum, 14*, 343–367.

Cole, T. R., Ray, R., & Kastenbaum, R. (2010). *A guide to humanistic studies in ageing*. Baltimore, MD: The Johns Hopkins University Press.

Coleman, A. (Ed.). (2000). *Jorge Luis Borges: Selected poems* (Two forms of insomnia). New York: Penguin Books.

Floridi, L. (2009). The information society and its philosophy: Introduction to the special issue on "philosophy of information, its nature, and future developments". *The Information Society, 25*, 153–158.

Goertzel, B. (2010). *AI against ageing—AIs, superflies, and the path to immortality*. Paper presented at the Singularity Summit, Hyatt Regency, San Francisco, CA. Retrieved August 14–15, 2010, from http://www.singularitysummit.com/abstracts/goertzel.

Graver, M. R. (2007). *Stoicism and emotion*. Chicago, IL: University of Chicago Press.

Hauskeller, M. (2010). Nietzsche, the overhuman and the posthuman: A reply to Stefan Sorgner. *Journal of Evolution & Technology, 21*(1), 5–8.

Hibbard, B. (2010). Nietzsche's overhuman is an ideal whereas posthumans will be real. *Journal of Evolution & Technology, 21*(1), 9–12.

Irvine, W. B. (2009). *A guide to the good life: The ancient art of stoic joy*. New York: Oxford University Press.

More, M. (2010). The overman in the transhuman. *Journal of Evolution & Technology, 21*(1), 1–4.

Pippin, R. B. (2010). *Nietzsche, psychology, & first philosophy*. Chicago: The University of Chicago Press.

Sorgner, S. L. (2009). Nietzsche, the overhuman, and transhumanism. *Journal of Evolution and Technology, 20*(1), 29–42.

Ure, M. (2009). Nietzsche's free spirit triology and stoic therapy. *Journal of Nietzsche Studies, 38*, 60–84.

Wicks, R. (2007). *Nietzsche*. Oxford: Oneworld Publications.

Index

K.F. Felsted and S.D. Wright, *Toward Post Ageing*,
Healthy Ageing and Longevity 1, DOI 10.1007/978-3-319-09051-1